UNSAFE
AT ANY
MEAL

OTHER BOOKS BY EARL MINDELL

Shaping Up With Vitamins
The Vitamin Bible

UNSAFE

AT ANY MEAL

Earl Mindell
R.Ph., Ph.D.

WARNER BOOKS

A Warner Communications Company

Warner Books, Inc., 666 Fifth Avenue, New York, NY 10103
W A Warner Communications Company

Printed in the United States of America

First Printing: April 1987

10 9 8 7 6 5 4 3 2 1

Library of Congress Cataloging-in-Publication Data

Mindell, Earl.
  Earl Mindell's unsafe at any meal.

  Bibliography: p. 226
  1. Food additives. 2. Food—Composition. I. Title.
II. Title: Unsafe at any meal.
TX553.A3M56 1987   613.2   86-40409
ISBN 0-446-51235-4

Book design: H. Roberts

This book is dedicated to Gail, Alanna, Evan, my parents and families, my friends and associates, and to the continuing happiness and healthiness of people everywhere.

Contents

1. The Lowdown on Labels   1

(1) Why you can't judge a food by its label—(2) What's allowed to go unmentioned is unforgivable—(3) "Labelese": How general terms can be particularly confusing—(4) Yes, what you don't know CAN harm you—(5) Basic "labelese" for beginners in search of better health—(6) The straight nutrition facts you are getting—(7) Check those serving sizes—(8) Where do those percentages come from? —(9) Becoming percentage wise—(10) How to find hidden ingredients—(11) Coping with invisible ingredients—(12) What's in a flavor?—(13) Flavoring labeling translated—(14) Those mysterious "spices"—(15) Are you getting the right USDA grades?—(16) Labels to double-check—(17) Any questions about Chapter 1?

2. Those Unpronounceable Additives   19

(18) What additives are—(19) Myth understanding—
(20) Unintentional additives—(21) The GRAS in your diet—
(22) Some popular GRAS additives you might want to keep off your shopping list—(23) What they do to your food—(24) What they can do to you: symptom-additive connections—(25) The new silent

Acknowledgments

I wish to express my deep and lasting appreciation to my friends and associates who have assisted me in the preparation of this book, especially J. Kenney, Ph.D.; Linus Pauling, Ph.D.; Harold Segal, Ph.D.; Bernard Bubman, R.Ph.; Mel Rich, R.Ph.; Sal Messineo, R.Ph.; Arnold Fox, M.D.; Dennis Huddleson, M.D.; Stewart Fisher, M.D.; Robert Mendelson, M.D.; Gershon Lesser, M.D.; David Velkoff, M.D.; Rory Jaffee, M.D.; Vickie Hufnagel, M.D.; Donald Cruden, O.D.; Joel Strom, D.D.S.; Nathan Sperling, D.D.S.; Rebecca Daniels; and Hester Mundis.

I would also like to thank the Nutrition Foundation; the International College of Applied Nutrition; the American Medical Association; the American Academy of Pediatrics; the American Dietetic Association; the National Academy of Sciences; the National Dairy Council; the Society for Nutrition Education; the United Fresh Fruit and Vegetable Association; the Albany College of Pharmacy; Betty Haskins; Ron Van Warmer; and Richard Curtis, without whose professional guidance and wise counsel this project could not have been successfully completed.

Preface

I find it ironic and frightening that today, when people are spending more money, time, and effort than ever before to learn how to shape up, eat to win, and keep fit for life, so few are aware of how much—and how often—their efforts are being nutritionally undermined. I can certainly understand why, but knowing the reason does not solve the problem. My hope is that this book will help to do that.

The problem is that a little bit of knowledge can be a dangerous thing, and lots of little bits can be even more dangerous. This is essentially what has happened. The public has been getting health information in nutritional bits and pieces. Snippets of facts about what foods are good for you and what ones aren't are tossed out like confetti, leaving consumers in a completely comprehensible state of confusion.

They are confused by unexplained factual contradictions (eggs are high in cholesterol yet can reduce the risk of heart disease), and vacillate between diametrically opposed diets (high-protein versus high-carbohydrate) to their own increasing detriment.

They are duped by deceptive advertising ("no preservatives" on labels of foods that contain them), victimized by government safety sanctions of potentially mutagenic, carcinogenic, and lethal additives (BHA, MSG, propyl gallate, etc.) and, in effect, are left unsafe at any meal.

As a consumer and parent, I recognized the need for a book that would explain clearly how, why, and what foods, additives, and environmental pollutants could adversely affect day-to-day fitness and shortchange lives. Being a nutritionist and pharmacist with lifetime dedication to spreading practical, health-promoting information and advice, I decided that when more than one-third of all children over the age of twelve have elevated cholesterol levels, when the average American consumes over 125 pounds of sugar and 15 pounds of salt annually without knowing it, when taking a 15-minute hot shower in L.A. is equivalent to drinking 8 glasses of contaminated water, and the "natural cheese" on a frozen pizza can be a chemical concoction of hazardous additives, this was a book that had to be written now.

The book has been designed as a realistic health-defense guide. I say realistic because I don't expect meat-loving readers to suddenly renounce charcoal-broiled steaks for tofu, or pretend that kids who are hooked on fast foods can be easily switched to whole grains. What I have done in many instances, though, is provide food trade-offs (lesser evils, so to speak) that can diminish health risks, and that *you* can live with—in more ways than one.

Each section is numbered and cross-referenced to help you easily locate information related to a particular food or additive. I've individualized, to the best of my ability, cautions pertaining to foods, drugs, and nutrients, by providing warning notices for high-risk consumers and alternatives for those who might have any medical problem or special health condition.

My supplement suggestions in *all* instances are *not* to be prescriptive. They are offered only as suggestions and should be discussed with your doctor. No book is or should be regarded as a substitute for professional care.

The primary purpose of this guide is to help you help yourself by understanding your own nutritional needs, how they are being met or undermined by what you're eating, and what health benefits you're really getting (or not getting) with every bite you take. I've also attempted to lift the grease curtain on convenience foods, fast foods, and foods you never thought were anything but wholesome; blow the whistle on seditious salt and sugar traps; shake you with the reality of deadly chemicals that might be pouring from your tap, hidden in your snacks, booze, "health food," breakfast, lunch, and dinner. I hope I've succeeded. When our top-selling cookies are made with slightly firm plastic material, and the government permits almost 3,000 additives to be hidden from consumers, it's time to spread the word—and get some changes made! It is my sincere desire that this book will do just that for all of you.

Earl L. Mindell, R.Ph., Ph.D.

Beverly Hills, California
September 1986

A Note to the Reader

The food and supplement regimens given throughout this book are *recommendations, not prescriptions, and are not intended as medical advice*. Before making any changes in your current diet or starting any supplement program, check with your physician or a nutritionally oriented doctor (see section 143), especially if you have a specific physical problem or are taking any medication.

All brand name nutritional information in the book is accurate as of December 1986.

1

THE LOWDOWN ON LABELS

1. Why You Can't Judge a Food by Its Label

Food labels are inadequate, confusing, and dangerously misleading sources of dietary information. In fact, at present the only labeling requirements for all foods are that they must: (a) tell what the product is and display its name on the main part of the label; (b) show the net weight or volume of the product; (c) give the name of the food manufacturer, packer, or distributor; and (d) list ingredients in descending order by weight.

This doesn't give you much to go on if you're counting calories, concerned about your protein intake, trying to avoid saturated fats, or sensitive to vegetable derivatives, spices, preservatives, and numerous other substances that need not appear on labels.

> Food labels are inadequate, confusing, and dangerously misleading sources of dietary information.

Nutrition information is essentially voluntary and is required *only* if a manufacturer makes a nutrition claim (for example, "high protein" or "low cholesterol"), or has added vitamins or minerals to fortify a product. Fortunately, if *any* nutritional information is given, *all* legally required information must appear on the product. Unfortunately, a lot of information is *not* legally required.

2. What's Allowed to Go Unmentioned Is Unforgivable

Considering that such auspicious agencies as the Departments of Agriculture and Commerce, the Food and Drug Administration, and the Federal Trade Commission are in charge of food labeling, it's unforgivable that:

• Specific identification of all flavorings, spices, fats, and oils is not required.
• Not all additives have to be listed.
• All products do not have to disclose the presence of specific artificial coloring unless the coloring has been *proven* hazardous to health (for instance, yellow dye FD&C No. 5, tartrazine).
• Sulfites, preservative chemicals implicated in more than a dozen deaths, do not have to be listed on all product labels.

I also think it's unforgivable that foods can legally claim "no preservatives" and still contain them because they are added before processing, that products labeled "salt free" can still have substantial amounts of sodium, but that's another story. It is called "labelese" and is about the deceptive-but-legal liberties manufacturers are allowed. It's not a pretty tale.

3. "Labelese": How General Terms Can Be Particularly Confusing

The Food and Drug Administration (FDA) and the United States Department of Agriculture (USDA) have established "Definitions" and "Standards of Identity" for food labeling. These regulations determine such things as minimum standards of composition for common foods, what additives need not be listed, when and what generalized terms may be used in place of specific ingredients.

What is considered safe today might not be tomorrow.

Their purpose—an admirable one—is to simplify label reading while protecting consumers from being ripped off, nutritionally and financially. It has resulted in more confusion than enlightenment for consumers—and more ways for manufacturers to hide ingredients that might make their product less appealing to buyers.

Though only safe ingredients are permitted for generalized categorization, what is safe for some people is not safe for all—and what is considered safe today might be proven otherwise tomorrow.

4. Yes, What You Don't Know CAN Harm You

Without a clear understanding of "labelese," you could be seriously undermining your health right now without knowing it.

Misinterpreting food label information can:

• Sabotage physical and emotional fitness
Cause fatigue, insomnia, headaches, stomachaches, nausea, rashes, diarrhea, dizziness, depression, mood swings, breathing difficulties, and more. (See section 24.)

• Decrease or alter the effectiveness of medications
Analgesics, antibiotics, anticoagulants, anticonvulsants, antidiabetics, antidyskinetics, antihistamines, antineoplastics, appetite suppressants, bronchial dilators, cardiovascular preparations, oral contraceptives, decongestants, diuretics, sedatives, thyroid drugs, tranquilizers, and more. (See section 126.)

5. Basic "Labelese" for Beginners in Search of Better Health

The following is a guide to the most commonly misinterpreted labels, explaining what they do—and do not—mean, and noting consumers who should be particularly aware of them.

LABELS MOST LIKELY TO MISLEAD

Diet or Dietetic

This simply means that the food contains no more than 40 calories *per serving*. It does NOT mean the food is necessarily low in sugar, sucrose, sodium, or even fat. Unless the label clearly states that the product is intended for use in a specific type of restricted diet, it generally isn't.

CONSUMER ALERT: Asthmatics, allergic individuals, hyperactive children.

Light or Lite

This usually means either one-third fewer calories than the regular product (which could have a lot more than you thought) or that it doesn't contain more than 40 calories per serving (which could be a lot less than you thought). But it can also mean lighter in syrup density, or color, or salt content. Though the label must state this, consumers don't often read the fine print and just assume that all light—or lite—products are low in calories.

CONSUMER ALERT: Dieters, hypertensives.

Light or Lean

When used on meat or poultry, whose labeling is regulated by the U.S. Department of Agriculture, this usually means a calorie reduction of 25 percent from the regular product (though it could be referring to something like breading or salt) and a comparison with the regular product must be given. Nonetheless, if you are concerned about your intake of fat, which you should be (no more than 20 percent of your daily calories should come from fat), you should be aware that those beguiling "lean" or "light" sausages still get about 70 percent of their calories from fat.

CONSUMER ALERT: Dieters, anyone with cardiovascular or gastrointestinal problems.

Light Beer or Wine

Labeling of beer and wine (see sections 77 to 80) is regulated by the Bureau of Alcohol, Tobacco, and Firearms (BATF). A light beer will usually have one-third fewer calories than its regular counterpart, but not always. Sometimes, the "light" refers to other factors, such as the beer's taste, color, or body. The same is basically true for wine. A "light" wine can contain no more than 14 percent alcohol, but then not many table wines do. And since there are no requirements for how few calories a "light" wine or beer contains, weight-watching consumers can be easily left in the dark.

CONSUMER ALERT: Dieters.

Low Calorie

A food labeled "low calorie" can have no more than 40 calories per serving. This is fair—it is the serving sizes that aren't. Because manufacturers can change them and do, what might formerly have been a single serving could now be two.

CONSUMER ALERT: Dieters.

Low Fat

On meat and poultry, whose labels are under USDA regulation, this means a product must have at least 25 percent less fat than a similar product. On foods whose labels are under FDA jurisdiction, which most packaged foods are, this can mean nothing. Because "low fat" has not yet been defined by FDA Standards of Identity, manufacturers are free to use the term at their discretion, which can dangerously mislead anyone concerned about their intake of cholesterol or calories.

CONSUMER ALERT: Dieters, anyone with cardiovascular or gastrointestinal problems.

Low Sodium

The product can have no more than 140 mg. per serving. This in itself is fine, but can mislead consumers who are unaware that former serving sizes might be nearly half their present ones, as is the case with many popular soups.

CONSUMER ALERT: Pregnant women, anyone with high blood pressure or cardiovascular problems.

No Artificial Flavors

Products so labeled can still contain artificial colors and preservatives, though most people assume them to be natural and free of all additives.

CONSUMER ALERT: Allergic individuals, pregnant and lactating women, hyperactive children.

Reduced Calorie

A product with one-third fewer calories per serving than it would have in its standard form. This can be very deceptive since the product can still have a higher caloric content than foods that are naturally low in calories.

CONSUMER ALERT: Dieters.

No Preservatives

Products that boast "no preservatives" can still contain them (they can be in the ingredients the manufacturer buys to make the products), as well as artificial colors and other additives.

CONSUMER ALERT: Allergic individuals, women who are pregnant or breast-feeding, hyperactive children.

No Cholesterol

Frequently used by manufacturers to make a product seem more nutritious—and worth paying more for—but virtually meaningless when used on foods of plant origin such as peanut butter or margarine, since the only foods with cholesterol are of animal origin. No cholesterol does *not* mean no fat! (Cholesterol is just one type of fat.)

CONSUMER ALERT: Cost-conscious shoppers, dieters.

Natural or All Natural

When used on a meat or poultry label, "natural" means that the product doesn't contain any artificial ingredients or chemical preservatives. But on other products, those whose labels are regulated by the FDA (most supermarket food), "natural" has no legal definition and is used by manufacturers to make people think the product is totally free of additives and chemicals—which is rarely, if ever, the case.

CONSUMER ALERT: Allergic individuals, women who are pregnant or breast-feeding, hyperactive children.

Naturally Sweetened

Once again, since "natural" has no legal FDA definition, calling a product "naturally sweetened" means little except for increasing sales. Be it honey, brown sugar, or corn syrup, a "naturally sweetened" product is neither necessarily lower in calories nor better for your health.

CONSUMER ALERT: Dieters, children.

Sodium Free

This does not mean the product is *free* of sodium, only that a serving has fewer than 5 mg.

CONSUMER ALERT: Anyone with high blood pressure or cardiovascular problems, pregnant women.

Unsalted, Salt Free, and No Salt Added

Though no salt was added during processing, "unsalted," "salt free," and "no salt added" products can still contain substantial amounts of sodium.

CONSUMER ALERT: Anyone with high blood pressure or cardiovascular problems, pregnant women.

Sugarless or Sugar Free

This means free of sugar (sucrose), but not other sweeteners (mannitol, sorbitol, and fructose, for example), and therefore such products can contain just as many calories as those with sugar. If so, the fine print must state this, or something to the effect of the product's usefulness only in not promoting tooth decay. Regrettably, not many buyers take the time to read the fine print.

CONSUMER ALERT: Dieters, anyone with gastrointestinal problems (mannitol and sorbitol can cause cramps, gas, bloating, and diarrhea).

Wheat Bread, Crackers, or Cereal

Manufacturers can present an image of whole wheat by calling a product "natural wheat" or "stone ground wheat," but unless "whole wheat" is first on the ingredient list you're not getting the whole truth—or whole wheat.

CONSUMER ALERT: Diabetics, dieters, anyone with gastrointestinal problems.

6. The Straight Nutrition Facts You Are Getting

According to FDA regulations, all nutrition information on food labels must:

• Be based on the U.S. Recommended Daily Allowance (U.S. RDA).
• Be given per serving.
• State serving size (in a recognizable household measure, such as cups, ounces, and tablespoons).
• State number of servings per container.
• State a serving's amount of calories, protein, carbohydrate, fat and sodium—in that specific order. (Cholesterol content may be given, but is not required.)
• Give the percentage of the U.S. Recommended Daily Allowance (see sections 8 and 9) supplied per serving by protein, vitamin A, vitamin C, thiamine, riboflavin, niacin, calcium, and iron—in

that specific order. (Twelve more vitamins and minerals for which a U.S. RDA has been established may be listed if a manufacturer so chooses; giving the percentage of calories from fat and amounts of fatty acids is also optional.)

• Show two columns of nutritive values for food normally combined with another food, such as breakfast cereal (which is usually combined with milk), giving percentages for the food in one column and the combination in the other.

7. Check Those Serving Sizes

Although nutrition information on food labels is given per serving, consumers frequently overlook serving sizes, an oversight that can get any *body* in trouble.

Unknown serving sizes can cause hefty portions of trouble.

Many a dieter has discovered this the hard way: by carefully counting calories and still putting on pounds. A 10½-ounce can of soup, for instance, might have only 70 calories a serving. But without checking the fine print for the manufacturer's serving size, *and* noting the servings per container (which are frequently more than you think), you're probably consuming almost double the number of calories you intended—particularly since all calories listed for a particular food are only averages. Now, twenty calories more or less might not sound like much. But just five foods containing twenty unlisted calories, eaten on a daily basis, can make you ten pounds heavier in a year. In ten years, that's one hundred pounds!

Keep in mind that manufacturers are allowed to determine how much *they* consider a serving, and will frequently reduce serving sizes to make products appear lower in calories, saturated fats, or sodium. So, what you assume is a serving and what a manufacturer says is a serving can be two different things—and very often are.

8. Where Do Those Percentages Come From?

The percentages of nutrients on food labels are based on the U.S.

RDA (Recommended Dietary Allowances), which in turn are based on the RDA. People frequently confuse the two, which are similar in that they both establish standards for nutrients.

RDA are determined and usually updated every five years by the Food and Nutrition Board of the National Research Council of the Academy of Sciences. They are *estimates* of nutritional needs to ensure satisfactory growth of children and the prevention of nutrient depletion in adults. *They are not meant to be optimal intakes, nor are they recommendations for an ideal diet.* They are not formulated to cover the needs of anyone who is ill, nor do they take into account nutrient losses that occur during food processing and preparation. They are recommendations intended to prevent deficiencies and meet the needs of *healthy* people with the highest requirements.

Just because a product contains 100 percent of the U.S. RDA for a nutrient, doesn't mean that you're getting it.

Even though the U.S. RDA are higher than the RDA, as far as many other nutritionists and I are concerned they are still inadequate. Individuals vary. Stress and illness, past or present, affect everyone's nutritional requirements differently. Just because a product claims to provide 100 percent of the U.S. RDA for a nutrient, doesn't necessarily mean that *you* are getting it, or that it's a sufficient amount for *your* individual needs—or even that the product actually contains 100 percent of that nutrient.

9. Becoming Percentage Wise
The FDA system for determining percentages of the U.S. RDA on food labels works like this:

IF A SERVING HAS...	THE PERCENTAGE IS...
More than 50 percent of the U.S. RDA for a nutrient	Shown to the nearest 10 percent
Between 10 and 50 percent of the U.S. RDA for a nutrient	Shown to the nearest 5 percent

IF A SERVING HAS . . .	THE PERCENTAGE IS . . .
Just 10 percent or less of the U.S. RDA for a nutrient	Shown to the nearest 2 percent
Less than 2 percent of the U.S. RDA for a nutrient	Shown as "0" or as an asterisk used with the footnote: "Contains less than 2 percent of the U.S. RDA of this nutrient (or these nutrients)."

If five or more nutrients are below 2 percent of the U.S. RDA, they do not have to be listed. But the manufacturer *can* use the footnote: "Contains less than 2 percent of the U.S. RDA of . . . (names of five or more nutrients)." For anyone just glancing quickly at the label, this could make even a candy bar appear nutritious.

10. How to Find Hidden Ingredients

The important thing to remember when looking at an ingredient panel is that the list is in decreasing order of quantity. In other words, you get the most of what comes first and the least of what comes last.

Sounds simple, right? Wrong. As anyone who has ever read a label knows, it's not so easy to figure out what a product contains even when the ingredients are listed. Right now, at least one hundred sweet substances are identified as sugars in products on the market, and manufacturers rely on the fact that the average consumer cannot identify them.

> It is not easy to figure out what a product contains even when the ingredients are listed.

Companies also count on consumers not being able to identify sodium, cholesterol, fats, and additives. But you can easily learn how, and the time to do it is now.

SPOT THOSE SUGARS

• Ingredients on labels ending in "-ose" indicate the presence of sugar. (For example, fructose is fruit sugar; dextrose, chemically identical to glucose, is made from cornstarch; maltose is malt sugar, formed from starch by yeast action; lactose is the sugar in milk.)

• Honey, corn syrup, corn syrup solids, maple syrup, molasses, and cane syrup, among over a hundred others, are also sugars.

SPOT THAT SALT

• Look for the words "salt" and "sodium" (either listed alone or in combinations such as sodium chloride, sodium stearoyl lactylate, sodium caseinate, and sodium citrate), and notice in what position (and how many times) they appear on the label.

• Watch for the chemical symbols Na and NaCl.

• Know that baking soda, baking powder, and MSG (monosodium glutamate) all spell salt.

• Be aware that products with shellfish (clams, lobster, shrimp) are naturally high in sodium. (See section 93 for sneaky high-salt foods.)

SPOT THAT SATURATED FAT

• Whether labeled "low fat" or "lean," packaged luncheon meats and hot dogs are still saturated with fat.

• If a label offers multiple-choice ingredients ("contains sunflower seed oil, coconut oil and/or palm oil"), and one is an unsaturated fat (sunflower seed oil) and the other(s) saturated, you are probably getting more saturated fat than you know.

• Though it comes in the guise of a liquid, whole milk is food with a whole lot of fat that a whole lot of people are not even aware of.

• Doughnuts and cakes, which most people just think of as sugar sources, can add a significant and potentially dangerous amount of fat to your diet.

11. Coping with Invisible Ingredients

When companies put labels on food they are responsible only for what *they* added to it. If they buy ingredients from manufacturers who have already presweetened, salted, or added additives to them, that need not be mentioned on the food label you see.

If you are concerned about your consumption of sugar or sodium or fat, it is important to always keep in mind that you're probably getting more of all three than you think.

YOUR BEST PROTECTION: Seek products with the least amounts of these ingredients, eat in moderation, and vary your diet. Remember that it is not necessarily *how much* sugar or salt or fat the food you eat contains but *how often* you eat foods containing them.

12. What's in a Flavor?

Let me put it this way: What you think you are tasting is probably not what you think you are tasting. If this sounds absurd, it's because it is. Natural flavors occur organically through the combining of many different natural chemicals. Once a flavor's basic composition is determined, laboratory scientists can concoct a facsimile "artificial flavoring" by isolating components from the natural source or synthesizing them chemically, and then adding whatever chemicals they want to create a more realistic (or economical) flavor.

> We consume hundreds of flavorings daily—and most have never even been tasted for safety.

Though the FDA is periodically informed of substances being used in flavorings, all a manufacturer has to do is declare (on the basis of minimal substantive testing) that a new artificial flavor is safe and it can be added to food without FDA approval or without listing the specific ingredients in the flavoring on the product label.

The frightening truth is that millions of us consume hundreds of flavorings daily—and most of them have never even been tested for their potential to cause cancer, birth defects, or any other health hazards.

13. Flavoring Labeling Translated

If a product does not actually *state* a flavor, such as "lemon" or "strawberry," or have a picture on the package that makes it look lemony or strawberryish, the manufacturer is allowed to list the ingredients as "natural flavors," "artificial flavors," or both.

This generalized and misleading information is unfair to all consumers and for some it is potentially dangerous. For example, undisclosed flavor ingredients could cause a variety of adverse reactions in sensitive individuals that might be mistakenly diagnosed and, if treated incorrectly, result in serious health complications.

Though flavor labeling says little, understanding it can help a lot.

IF THE LABEL SAYS...	THE PRODUCT HAS...
Strawberry pudding	Only natural strawberry flavor (which must come entirely from strawberries)
Strawberry pudding with other natural flavors	Strawberries and another natural characterizing flavor (strawberry extract, for example)
Strawberry-flavored pudding	More natural than added artificial flavoring
Artificially flavored strawberry pudding	Either all artificial flavoring or mostly artificial flavoring

FOOD FOR THOUGHT: The FDA Register states than "an artificial flavor is no less safe, no less nutritious, and not inherently less desirable than a natural flavor." In all cases? Not in my book!

14. Those Mysterious "Spices"

> Just because spices occur naturally does not mean that they can't harm you.

Have you ever wondered what those nameless "spices" on ingredient labels are? It's not surprising since they can be one or more of dozens that need not be listed because—by FDA designation—they are aromatic vegetable substances that season and have no nutritional value. If the spice adds color, as in the case of paprika, turmeric, and saffron, it must either be listed by name or as "spice and coloring." Only garlic, onion, and celery seasoning, because they are considered food, must be specifically identified.

This sort of ambiguous labeling can be dangerous, especially for the more than 30 million Americans who are allergic to the tiniest amount of certain chemicals. Simply because most spices occur naturally, and relatively small amounts of them are used in a food, does not mean they can't harm you. Nor does long use ensure safety. Safrole, which cames from sassafras, was used to flavor root beer for years before it was discovered to cause liver cancer.

15. Are You Getting the Right USDA Grades?

The USDA is responsible for inspecting and grading meats, poultry, fresh fruits and vegetables, eggs, and most dairy products. The grading and quality marks are based essentially on little more than certain standards of cleanliness necessary for public health safety, and offer virtually no clue to the food's nutritive value.

But as inadequate as USDA grading is, it can at least provide you with some indication of a food's quality. Also, by recognizing government marks, you're less likely to be fooled by private gradings, which are used in many stores to disguise inferior meats and poultry.

WHAT TO WATCH OUT FOR

When buying fresh fruits and vegetables: Be wary of crates without government stamps, such as "U.S. Grade No. 1," or that are not marked "Packed Under Continuous Inspection of the U.S. Department of Agriculture" or "Packed by [name of company] Under Continuous Federal-State Inspection."

When buying poultry: Watch out for the lack of a state or federal inspection stamp (that is, "Inspected for Wholesomeness by U.S. Department of Agriculture P-42"), or a "USDA A Grade" stamp, which indicates quality. (Birds below "A" grade are often privately labeled "Premium" or "Quality" by store owners, so beware.)

When buying meats: Avoid any that are not stamped with the abbreviation "U.S. INSP'D & P'S'D." Meat that crosses state lines must be inspected for cleanliness. The mark is not on each cut, but should be on each carcass. (You can ask the store manager to show you the stamped carcass if you want to be sure you are buying safe meat.) Quality grading (i.e. fat and marbling content; highest deemed "prime") is done at the packer's request, and each cut of meat is stamped ("Prime," "Choice," "Good," "Standard," or "Commercial"). Meats below "Choice" are not likely to sell well, so markets will often supply their own grades, such as "Excellent" or "Top Quality." Canned, frozen, dried, or packaged meat products should have an inspection mark (that is, "U.S. INSPECTED AND PASSED BY DEPARTMENT OF AGRICULTURE EST. 38") to show that the food is sanitary and the label has been approved by the USDA for truthfulness.

When buying milk: Avoid any that is not "Grade A" and pasteurized. Raw milk has more vitamin C than processed milk, but since milk is not a prime source of vitamin C, the risk of illness (cattle disease and tuberculosis can be transmitted to people through raw milk) outweighs its benefits.

16. Labels to Double-Check
Computerized market research has enabled food advertising and packaging to reach frighteningly effective heights, but at a great expense—your health. Reread section 10 and carefully scrutinize the ingredients (and their order of appearance on the label) of any foods that claim:

• They are nutritionally superior to competing brands or similar whole foods.
• They can help you control appetite and lose weight.
• They supply your complete requirement for all or any nutrients.
• They can improve health or prevent disease.

17. Any Questions About Chapter 1?
Does the "net" weight of a canned product mean the actual weight of the food without the liquid it's packed in?
The use of the word "net" might make it appear that way ("net

income," after all, means what you actually have after deductions), but the answer is no. The net weight on labels means everything— water, syrup, oil—that is contained along with the food in the can, jar, or package. The only thing deducted is the weight of the container.

One 6½-ounce can of tunafish, for instance, might be more expensive than another brand, yet still contain less tuna.

I'm very confused by the weights and measures used on most product labels. Do you have some sort of simple guide that can help an old shopper figure out how new foods measure up?

The terminology is really less confusing than you think. The metric system is used for most RDA measurements of nutrients, and they are measured in very small amounts by weight—grams (g.), milligrams (mg.), micrograms (mcg. or ug.), etc.

For fat-soluble vitamins (A, E, D, and K) the system of measurement is International Units (IU). IU measures the biological activity of a nutrient (its ability to support growth) rather than weight. Vitamin A values, though, are now also given in retinol equivalents (RE)—that is, the equivalent weight of retinol (vitamin A_1, alcohol) *actually absorbed and converted*. Retinol equivalents come out to be about five to fifteen times less than International Units. In the case of vitamin A, an RDA of 5,000 IU would be the same as 1,000 RE.

But if that's more than you wanted to know, the following conversions should help:

QUICKIE CONSUMER CONVERSIONS

1 kilogram = 1,000 grams (g.) = 2.2 pounds (lb.)
1 pound   = 16 ounces (oz.)
1 ounce   = 28 grams   = 2 tablespoons (tbsp.)
1 gram   = 1,000 milligrams (mg.)
1 milligram = 1,000 micrograms (mcg. or ug.)
1 gallon   = 4 quarts
1 quart   = 2 pints   = 32 fluid ounces (fl. oz.)
1 pint   = 2 cups
1 cup   = 8 ounces
½ cup   = 8 tablespoons (liquid) and 6 tablespoons (dry)

What does "imitation" margarine or mayonnaise mean?

It means the product isn't the real thing, and is also nutritionally inferior—lower in nutrients. (That doesn't mean, necessarily, lower in fat, calories, or cholesterol.) If it is nutritionally on a par with the food it is copying, the term "substitute" may be used—or the product can have a name implying that it is what it is not. For example, such wording as "spreadable Peanut Swirl" can be used for an imitation peanut butter that has the same nutrient value as the real thing. That way neither the word "imitation" nor "substitute" need appear on the label.

Is a food labeled "organic" better than one labeled "natural"?

It depends on the ingredients because neither "organic" nor "natural" has a legal FDA definition. Manufacturers may use either or both terms at their discretion—which usually leaves much to be desired.

2

THOSE UNPRONOUNCEABLE ADDITIVES

18. What Additives Are

Additives are substances other than basic ingredients that are added to foods for numerous reasons; some of them praiseworthy, some appallingly not.

On the praiseworthy side, they are used to increase flavor, improve nutritional value, retard spoilage, extend shelf life, simplify preparation, and make more products readily available to consumers. On the other hand, they are used as adulterants to disguise inferior foods with dangerous dyes and chemicals so that manufacturers can make higher profits. (There are laws against this, of course, but they are difficult to enforce.)

An additive can be a naturally occurring food substance, such as vinegar (acetic acid), a chemical concoction such as BHA (butylated hydroxyanisole), or a combination of both (most artificial food flavors), but to qualify for usage it must meet three FDA requirements:

- Perform a useful function in the food.
- Be safe for human consumption even if eaten in excessively large amounts over a lifetime.
- Not contribute to the growth of cancer in test animals, even when the amounts fed in laboratory tests are in excess of any amount possible for a human to consume in a lifetime.

Before any new additive may be used, it must be extensively tested for toxicity on animals. The only catch is that the manufacturer, not the FDA, does the testing.

19. Myth Understanding

Considering that the average person consumes more than 4 pounds of food additives each year, it's unbelievable how little is understood by so many about so much.

ADDITIVE MYTHS

• All additives are bad.
(All additives are not bad—at least not *all bad*. For instance, most preservatives used to prevent the growth of bacteria that cause deadly botulism offer benefits that outweigh their risks.)
• Some additives are completely safe.
(No additive is completely safe for all people all of the time. The most innocuous additives—even ordinary foods, for that matter—are capable of causing adverse reactions during illness, for example, or if ingested while taking certain medications. Also, substances that are harmless for adults can be dangerous for children.)
• Foods in the old days were safer and more wholesome.
(Foods have been adulterated for centuries. Two hundred years ago more dangerous additives were used than today. In fact, popular sugar confections contained mineral dyes that killed people every year.)
• Natural additives are safer than chemical ones.
(Not necessarily. Coumarin, from tonka beans, was used for seventy-five years in flavorings before it was found to cause liver damage.)
• Naturally preserved meats are safe and chemical free.
(Whether done in old smokehouses or new factories, the smoking process produces resinous, cancer-causing chemicals that are imparted to the food.)

20. Unintentional Additives

Numerous manufacturing contaminants (detergents, solvents, lubricating oils, textile fibers, plastics, and so forth), used in the production, storage, and transportation of partially prepared foods or ingredients, often wind up in the final product. But because they weren't *intended* to be there, they don't have to be mentioned on labels.

Unintentional additives can go unmentioned.

The same is true for antibiotics, hormones, and pesticides, whose residues not only can enter our foods, but also remain active even after cooking and digestion.

This is particularly distressing since more than 2 billion pounds of highly toxic and potentially carcinogenic pesticides are used annually by farmers, and only 100 of 600 insecticide ingredients in use have been reviewed for safety by the Environmental Protection Agency (EPA). Moreover, only four of these have been completely tested for their toxic effects on humans, and their long-term health hazards are still unknown.

21. The GRAS in Your Diet

Just because an additive has been declared GRAS (Generally Recognized As Safe) doesn't mean that it can't harm you. When the food additive law requiring scientific testing of all chemicals for safe usage in foods went into effect in 1958, the FDA established the GRAS list to eliminate expensive testing of what were unquestionably assumed to be safe chemicals (sugar, starch, salt, baking soda, etc.). By doing this, all additives in use before 1958 were deemed GRAS; unfortunately, quite a few were later found to be otherwise.

Though most of these have been removed from the list, many of questionable safety remain, posing dangers that no one can afford to ignore. Think about these:

• GRAS additives have more liberal limits on concentrations at which they may be added to foods, and the foods to which they may be added.

• GRAS additives, unlike others, can be used by manufacturers *without prior FDA approval*. Such usage might later be challenged by the FDA, but that is no consolation if your health has been irrevocably damaged.

• GRAS additives, because they are assumed to be harmless, are consumed in quantity and without question, and can therefore jeopardize the well-being of countless unwary individuals.

22. Some Popular GRAS Additives You Might Want to Keep Off Your Shopping List

ACACIA GUM (Gum Arabic)

Possible Adverse Effects Mild to severe asthma attacks, rashes; has caused fatalities in pregnant animals.

High-risk Individuals Anyone prone to allergies, asthmatics, pregnant women.

Prime Product Sources Soft candies, hard candies, frostings, chewing gum, soft drinks. (See section 74 for safer trade-offs.)

MY ADVICE: There is a possibility that this additive may have mutagenic or teratogenic (abnormal embryo development) properties. If you're pregnant, trying to become pregnant, or a nursing mother, avoid products containing acacia or similar vegetable gums, particularly carrageenan (used frequently in chocolate products, chocolate-flavored drinks, pressure-dispensed whipped cream, beverages, puddings, and syrups), gum tragacanth (fruit jellies, sherbets, and salad dressings), and carob or locust bean gum (flavorings for beverages, ice cream, baked goods, and gelatin desserts).

ALGINIC ACID

Possible Adverse Effects Pregnancy complications, birth defects; has caused maternal and fetal deaths in animals.

High-risk Individuals Pregnant or lactating women.

Prime Product Sources Ice cream, ice milk, fruit sherbet, frozen custards, cheese spreads, salad dressings.

MY ADVICE: Alginic acid (which, by the way, is also used in the manufacture of textiles, artificial ivory, and glue) is still being investigated as a possible mutagen, capable of causing reproductive problems and birth defects. If you're pregnant, trying to conceive, or a nursing mother, limiting your intake of products containing this GRAS additive or other alginates (ammonium/calcium/potassium/ sodium alginate; propylene glycol alginate; algin gum; algin derivatives) is highly recommended.

B E N Z O I C   A C I D

Possible Adverse Effects
Gastrointestinal irritation, asthma attacks, rashes, itching, irritation of eyes and mucous membranes neurological disorders, hyperactivity in children.

High-risk Individuals
Anyone prone to allergies, asthmatics, young children, people with liver problems.

Prime Product Sources
Jelly, jams, fruit juices, margarine, beer, pickles, bottled soft drinks, Maraschino cherries, marinated herring, mincemeat, barbecue sauce.

MY ADVICE: Despite GRAS status, benzoic acid and its salt sodium benzoate have been implicated in causing hyperactivity in children and mild to severe reactions in allergic individuals; for dogs and cats, 2 grams are lethal. Since this preservative combines with glycine in the liver, increasing that organ's workload, anyone with cirrhosis, hepatitis, or other liver ailment should consult a physician before consuming products containing benzoate additives.

B H A (Butylated hydroxyanisole)
and
B H T (Butylated hydroxytoluene)

Possible Adverse Effects
Elevated cholesterol levels, allergic reactions, liver damage, kidney damage, infertility, sterility, behavioral problems, loss of vitamin D, weakened immune system, increased susceptibility to cancer-causing substances.

High-risk Individuals	Infants, young children, pregnant or lactating women, anyone with allergies, heart, liver, or kidney problems, asthmatics.
Prime Product Sources	Chewing gum, candy, instant potato flakes, breakfast cereals, gelatin, desserts, dry mixes for desserts and beverages, lard, shortenings, unsmoked dry sausage, freeze-dried meats.

MY ADVICE: Both BHA and BHT have been found to affect liver and kidney functions. Though BHA has been shown to be less toxic than BHT, both are possible carcinogens, causes of allergic reactions, have potential mutagenic properties, and should be avoided by high-risk individuals as much as possible.

CAFFEINE
(See section 42)

GLUTAMIC ACID (Glutamic acid hydrochloride, monammonium, monopotassium, monosodium glutamate—MSG)

Possible Adverse Effects	Allergic reactions (particularly burning sensations, facial and chest pressure, and headaches), eye inflammations, brain edema (excessive fluid retention), central nervous and vascular system problems.
High-risk Individuals	Infants and young children, anyone with high blood pressure or other cardiovascular problems, anyone with allergies, particularly to sugar beets, corn, or wheat, pregnant women.
Prime Product Sources	Chinese food, sodium-free salt substitutes, seasoning salts, soups, condiments, pork sausages.

MY ADVICE: Glutamic acid and its salts are no longer being added to infant foods, as well they shouldn't be. Foods containing glutamates should be avoided, or at least limited in their intake, by all children. Decreases in brain function and learning abilities have occurred in test animals. If you have an eye inflammation—or are preparing to have any eye surgery—keep glutamates out of your diet. Also be aware that if you have high blood pressure, glutamic acids can weaken the protective blood-brain barrier, the membrane surrounding the brain, causing unwanted excitability. And since the placenta concentrates MSG, doubling the amount the fetus is exposed to, it's wise for pregnant women to limit their intake until further testing is completed.

IRON SALTS
(Ferric pyrophosphate, ferric sodium pyrophosphate, ferrous lactate)

Possible Adverse Effects   Gastrointestinal disturbances, tumors.

High-risk Individuals   Anyone with hemochromatosis, ulcers, pregnant women.

Prime Product Sources   Enriched bread, breakfast cereals, poultry, stuffing, self-rising flours, farina, cornmeal.

MY ADVICE: There has been limited and insufficient testing of the long-term and carcinogenic properties of these additives. There is no need for you or any member of your family to be a guinea pig; avoid these particular iron salts when possible.

PROPYL GALLATE

Possible Adverse Effects   Gastric irritation, asthmatic reactions, reproductive failures, liver and kidney damage, allergic reactions.

High-risk Individuals   Asthmatics, anyone with liver problems, children, anyone allergic to aspirin, pregnant women.

Prime Product Sources   Vegetable oils and shortenings, dry
breakfast cereals, flavorings for beverages, snack
foods, candies, gum, frozen dairy products.

MY ADVICE: Since propyl gallate is frequently used in combination with BHA and BHT, it can intensify the problems caused by those additives. Its potential carcinogenic and gene-altering properties have not been sufficiently tested, so I'd suggest waiting until they have before ingesting large amounts of it. It has been banned from foods intended for babies and young children in England.

23. What They Do to Your Food

Additives have numerous functions, and almost as many terms and categories to explain them. The following are those most commonly seen, heard, and misunderstood:

ACIDS

Substances used frequently in many processed foods, particularly in breads and other baked goods to cause the desired "rising" (potassium acid tartrate, sodium aluminum phosphate, tartaric acid); in soft drinks to modify flavor (citric acid, malic acid, tartaric acid, phosphoric acid); in butter to help preserve flavor and retard spoilage (usually the same acids that are used in soft drinks).

ALKALIES

Used to neutralize excess acidity in such foods as cocoa products, candies, cookies, and crackers (ammonium hydroxide, ammonium carbonate).

ANTIOXIDANTS

Preservatives for fats and oils to prevent rancidity and the development of off-flavors that can cause sickness. Used in margarine, shortenings, lard, soup stocks, dehydrated potatoes, potato chips, salted peanuts, cheese spreads, and many more products (benzoic acid, BHA, BHT). Also, since oxygen activates enzymes that tend to discolor cut fruits and vegetables, and make them less salable, antioxidants such as sodium sulfite, ascorbic acid, and sulfur dioxide are used on these, too. (See section 26 on sulfites.)

ANTISTALING AGENTS

Used to prevent crystallization of starch, which makes bread turn stale, hard, and unsalable, these are called bread emulsifiers but are actually antifirming agents (mono- and diglycerides, diacetyl tartaric acid esters of mono- and diglycerides, succinylated mono- and diglycerides).

BLEACHING AND MATURING AGENTS

For improving the baking quality of flour by accelerating its oxidation while also functioning as yeast foods and dough conditioners (potassium bromate, potassium iodate, calcium peroxide, ammonium or calcium sulfate salts, ammonium phosphates).

BUFFERS

Added to processed foods to control acidity or alkalinity (ammonium bicarbonate, calcium carbonate, potassium acid tartrate, sodium aluminum phosphate, tartaric acid).

DOUGH CONDITIONERS

Used in breads and baked goods to produce uniformity, despite variations in flour quality, by making dough drier and easier to work with (calcium stearyl-2-lactylate, sodium stearyl fumarate).

EMULSIFIERS

Widely used in margarines, shortenings, ice cream, baked goods, and many other processed foods to perform the formerly impossible mixing—without separation—of water in oil (mono- and diglycerides, sorbitan monostearate), and oil in water (polysorbates, polyoxyethylene sorbitan fatty acid esters), to provide uniform smoothness and homogeneity. Lecithin, from egg yolks, is the most widely used natural emulsifier (it is in the federal Standards of Identity for mayonnaise), though lecithin from soybeans is being used more frequently in non-standardized products.

EXCIPIENTS

Carrier substances for additives used in bread. A pharmacological term for any inactive substance used to bind an active one into a form for usage.

EXTRACTS

The result of passing alcohol or alcohol-and-water through natural essences, such as lemon, orange, banana, and vanilla. As flavoring solutions, they are known as extracts and can be purchased in supermarkets for home use. Since they are often too weak for effective flavoring, their potency is allowed to be intensified by combining them with other natural flavors. But the extract must contain at least 51 percent of the original fruit's flavor to be labeled as its extract.

FLAVOR ENHANCERS OR MODIFIERS

Substances with virtually no flavor of their own that are used in soups, sauces, cheeses, and products containing meat, poultry, seafood, and other protein, to maximize flavor without having to increase the amount or quality of the product's ingredients (monosodium glutamate [MSG], see section 22). Also used for intensifying flavor in chocolate, vanilla, and fruit-flavored foods and beverages, such as gelatin desserts, soft drinks, and other high carbohydrate products, as well as to mask bitter aftertaste in diet foods and lower the sugar content of regular foods (maltol, ethyl maltol).

HUMECTANTS

Moisture-control substances used to prevent foods, particularly icings, candy, and other confections, from drying out (glycerine, propylene glycol, sorbitol) and to prevent table salt from caking (calcium silicate).

LEAVENING AGENTS

Used in bread and other bakery products to keep them light and obtain desired rising (mostly phosphates, such as monocalcium, dicalcium, sodium acid, and sodium aluminum phosphate, but also acids, which are mentioned above).

NATURAL AND ARTIFICIAL COLORING

Contained in virtually all our processed foods in one form or the other (often both), color additives are used to keep foods looking the way consumers have been led to believe they should look—even if that is not the way they really do look. For example, oranges are actually green (see section 33), but that's not the color we have been taught oranges ought to be, and few consumers would buy them that way. They would be even more reluctant to purchase foods that, without additive dyes, would discolor after processing and storage. Colorings can also make products appear to contain ingredients that, in fact, they don't. And aside from being implicated in serious, adverse physical and emotional reactions in susceptible individuals, many government-certified colorings used in popular foods have been shown to be cancer-causing substances. (For more on natural and artificial colorings, see section 72.)

NATURAL AND ARTIFICIAL FLAVORINGS

All flavor additives are used to achieve long-lasting, uniform, consumer-preferred product tastes. They potentiate desired flavors, conceal undesirable ones, and even create some (artificial bacon bits, for instance, which are made from soybean protein). Natural extracts, essential oils (highly concentrated flavors obtained from fruit rinds), spices, oleoresins (concentrated spice extracts), and combinations of synthetic and natural substances are used as flavor additives in hundreds of processed foods, particularly soft drinks, ice cream, baked goods, confections, syrups, margarines, and shortenings (ethyl acetate, propionate, maloneate, and butyrate; caproic acid; decylaldehyde; diacetyl).

NEUTRALIZING AGENTS

Function the same as buffers.

POLYSORBATES

Emulsifiers (see p. 28) used to enhance the freezing qualities of ice cream and improve the texture of cake mixes (polyethylene [20], polysorbate [60], polysorbate [80]).

PRESERVATIVES

Used to prevent the growth of microorganisms and help prevent spoilage and mold in virtually all processed foods. In bread, they are used primarily to extend shelf life and prevent mold (acetic acid, lactic acid, sodium and calcium propionate, sodium diacetate), as they are in cheeses, canned pie fillings, and syrups (sodium and potassium salts, sorbic acid). Because of their versatility, the most widely used preservatives are propyl gallate, sulfur dioxide, sugar, salt, and vinegar.

PROPELLANTS

Gases or easily vaporized liquids used as whipping agents for dessert toppings and to expel contents of other foods, such as processed cheeses and icings, that are sold in aerosol containers (nitrogen, carbon dioxide, nitrous oxide).

SEQUESTRANTS

Preservatives to prevent physical or chemical changes, caused by trace metals, that adversely affect the flavor, texture, or appearance of food, such as the premature setting of dessert mixes, discoloration of canned foods, and the clouding of soft drinks (EDTA—ethylenediaminetetraacetic acid—salts), as well as the loss of freshness and sweetness in dairy products (calcium, potassium, and sodium salts of citric, tartaric, and pyrophosphoric acids).

As sequestrants, EDTA salts are also used in beer to control the suds spritz that occurs when a can or bottle is opened.

STABILIZERS AND TEXTURIZERS

These function much like emulsifiers, leavening agents, and thickeners. They keep ice cream consistently smooth and creamy by preventing water from freezing into grainy crystals. They also retard the settling of particles in liquid diet foods (eliminating the need to "shake well before using"), the cocoa particles in chocolate drinks, and the pulp particles in orange drinks, as well as improve the foaming properties of brewed beer (carrageenan, gelatin, carob bean gum, agar-agar, methylcellulose).

In cured meats, they are used to stabilize the pink color (sodium nitrate, sodium nitrite. See section 35).

SURFACTANTS

These fall into numerous categories, such as emulsifiers, foaming agents, stabilizers, and more. They're used in peanut butter, for instance, to keep oil and water mixtures from separating; in salad dressings they're used as thickeners. (Cellulose derivatives and vegetable gums are often classified as surfactants.)

SYNERGISTS

Substances capable of increasing the effect of another substance. Used to enhance the effects of antioxidant additives (citric and tartaric acid; calcium, potassium, and sodium salts).

THICKENERS

Like stabilizers, emulsifiers, leavening agents, and other texturizers, they are used to improve or maintain a product's desired body and consistency. They increase the firmness of canned tomatoes (amounts standardized by the FDA), potatoes, and sliced apples to prevent them from falling apart (calcium chloride, calcium citrate, mono- and dicalcium phosphate).

In artificially sweetened soft drinks, they're used to replace the body and thickness that would ordinarily be contributed by sugar. And in cheese spreads, gravies, icings, pie fillings, salad dressing, and syrups, they create any desired consistency (sodium alginate, pectins, natural vegetable gums which also work as stabilizers).

24. What They Can Do to You: Symptom-Additive Connections

Additive side effects are more common than most people (and many doctors) imagine, but they are usually assumed to be symptoms of other diseases—and treated as such. This is easy to understand, since Swiss cheese sandwiches for lunch would seem unlikely to be responsible for your migraines—but they could be! The same holds true for other discomforts, such as mouth or eye pains, which frequently send people off to dentists and ophthalmologists for medications they don't need.

Obviously, a doctor should always be consulted if any condition is causing consternation; but before rushing and getting a prescription (which is likely to have its own side effects), look over the following list and see if there is any relationship between the way you feel and the food additives you're eating—and then be sure to discuss these with your doctor. (*This list is by no means all-inclusive, but it should give you a pretty good idea of the numerous symptom-additive connections there can be.*)

SYMPTOM	POSSIBLE ADDITIVE CULPRIT
Anemia	Potassium nitrite
Asthma (breathing problems)	Acacia (gum arabic); acetal; allyl sulfide; benzoic acid; potassium nitrite; propyl gallate (all gallates); sodium nitrite; sodium, potassium, and calcium benzoate; sodium sulfite (and all other sulfites); tartrazine (or other azo or "coal tar" dyes)
Blurred vision	Tartrazine (or other azo dyes)
Constipation	Aluminum hydroxide
Depression	Benzaldehyde; benzyl alcohol; butyl acetate
Diarrhea	Acetic acid; benzyl alcohol; calcium disodium EDTA; capsicum (cayenne pepper); L-ascorbic acid (vitamin C); mannitol; monopotassium glutamate; potassium bromate; sorbitol; sorbitol syrup
Dizziness	MSG; sodium and other nitrites
Edema (retention of fluid)	Sodium acetate; synthetic "coal tar" or azo dyes
Elevated blood sugar	Glycerol
Excessive thirst	Glycerol

SYMPTOM	POSSIBLE ADDITIVE CULPRIT
Eye irritant	Acetic acid; biphenyl (diphenyl); butyl acetate; cornstarch
Faintness	MSG; potassium metabisulfite (potassium prosulfite)
Flatulence and bloating	Agar-agar; guar gum; pectin; sorbitol; sorbitol syrup
Flushing	Aluminum nicotinate; nicotinic acid (niacin nicotinamide)
Gastrointestinal upset or pain	Acetic acid; aloe extract; aluminum nicotinate; aluminum potassium sulfate; ammonium chloride; ammonium hydrogen carbonate (ammonium bicarbonate); benzoic acid; calcium chloride; calcium disodium EDTA; calcium gluconate; capsicum (cayenne pepper); guar gum; monopotassium glutamate; polyoxyethylene stearates; potassium bromate; potassium chloride; potassium hydroxide; potassium nitrate; propyl gallate; sodium and potassium polyphosphates; sodium carbonate; sodium metabisulfite (and all sulfites); synthetic "coal tar" or azo dyes; tartaric acid
Hay fever	Cornstarch; tartrazine (or other azo dyes)
Headaches	Glycerol; MSG; sodium nitrite and other nitrites; sodium propionate
Heart problems	Acetal; calcium chloride; calcium gluconate; coconut oil; sodium carbonate; sodium sulfate

SYMPTOM	POSSIBLE ADDITIVE CULPRIT
High blood pressure	Acetal; Indigo Carmine (or other "coal tar" dyes); MSG
Inflamed or ulcerated colon	Carrageenan
Inflammation of the tongue	Caramel
Itching	FD&C Blue No. 1 and 2 (or other "coal tar" or azo dyes); MSG
Kidney problems	Aloe extract; allyl sulfide; ammonium chloride; bromated vegetable oils; EDTA; L-ascorbic acid (in large doses); magnesium sulfate (epsom salts); polyoxyethylene stearates; potassium acetate; sodium sulfate
Liver problems	Allyl sulfide; ammonium chloride; propyl gallate (and all alkyl gallates)
Low blood pressure	FD&C Blue No. 1 and 2 (or other "coal tar" or azo dyes); MSG
Mouth ulcers or burning sensation in mouth	Aluminum, ammonium, or potassium sulfate; anethole; potassium hydroxide; tripotassium citrate (potassium citrate)
Nausea	Ammonium and potassium chloride; biphenyl (diphenyl); glycerol; guar gum; mannitol; monopotassium glutamate; MSG; sodium and other nitrites; synthetic "coal tar" or azo dyes
Nose irritant	Biphenyl (diphenyl); cornstarch
Overactive thyroid function	Erythrosine (a "coal tar" dye)

Symptom	Possible Additive Culprit
Purple patches on skin	Tartrazine (or other azo dyes)
Raised cholesterol levels	BHA; BHT
Reproductive failure	BHT; cedar leaf oil
Scalp lesions, crusts, dandruff, hair loss	Caramel
Sensitivity to light	Angelica; bergamot; cedar leaf oil; clover; erythrosine (a "coal tar" dye)
Skin rashes	Acacia (gum arabic); acetic acid; alkyl sulfates; benzoic acid; benzoyl peroxide; cinnamon bark extract and oil; polyoxyethylene stearates; sodium, potassium, and calcium benzoate; sodium metabisulfite (and other sulfites); sorbic acid; tartrazine (or other azo or "coal tar" dyes)
Tooth or gum erosion	Citric acid
Urinary disorders	Ammonium chloride; EDTA; formic acid; sodium and calcium formate; polyoxyethylene stearates
Vomiting	Acetic acid; aluminum ammonium sulfate; ammonium and potassium chloride; benzyl alcohol; biphenyl (diphenyl); calcium disodium EDTA; chamomile; mannitol; monopotassium glutamate; potassium bromate; potassium hydroxide; sodium and other nitrites; synthetic "coal tar" or azo dyes

25. The New Silent Additive

It is called irradiation. You don't smell it; you don't taste it. But it's classified as an additive by the FDA, is being readied for use on fresh fruits and vegetables, and has not yet been proven conclusively safe for human consumption!

For over twenty years, irradiation (a "cold sterilization" process involving gamma rays and high-energy electrons), has been used to kill insects in wheat and flour and control microbial contamination of spices and seasonings, as well as to destroy trichina parasites in pork—but not without taking its toll.

According to Public Citizen, a consumer advocate organization that has investigated studies done on irradiation:

• Only 1 percent of all studies reviewed appeared to support safety.

• Food exposed to the same levels of radiation being proposed for use on consumer poultry and meats caused testicular tumors in mice, and significantly reduced life expectancy in other laboratory test groups.

• Malnourished children who consumed freshly irradiated wheat had an increase in abnormal white blood cells.

• The current FDA proposal exempts irradiated fruits and vegetables exposed to less than the proposed 100 kilorads of radiation (which could mean 99) from all toxicological testing!

The Department of Health and Human Services refers to irradiated food as "picowaved" (sounds like microwaved, which is less threatening to consumers) and wanted this word used to label irradiated foods. To their credit, the USDA rejected it.

On the other hand, "Picofresh" has already been approved as a brand name for irradiated pork—which means more "pico" foods may soon be coming down the pike. Just something to keep in mind.

26. The Sinister Six Sulfites

They have been removed from the GRAS list and banned from use on fresh produce and cut fruits and vegetables, but many supermarkets, restaurants, and salad bars continue to use them. They function as sanitary agents and preservatives to help prevent the discoloration of dehydrated, frozen, and fermented fruits and vegetables. They keep potatoes white and lettuce green, and they have been implicated in the deaths of thirteen persons.

Collectively they are known as sulfiting agents and go under the following names on ingredient listings:

- potassium bisulfite
- sodium bisulfite
- sodium sulfite
- potassium metabisulfite
- sodium metabisulfite
- sulfur dioxide

If you're asthmatic, prone to allergies, or deficient in the liver enzyme sulfite oxidase, they can kill you!

At present, these additives are banned from use only on fresh fruits and vegetables, and are considered safe for *healthy* individuals who don't excessively consume foods or beverages in which they are present. The trouble is, they are excessively present. (See section 28.)

Reactions in sulfite-sensitive individuals can range from mild breathing difficulties to anaphylactic shock. Symptoms may include severe headaches, faintness, abdominal pains, nasal stuffiness, facial flushing, and diarrhea, either singly or in any possible combination. These reactions, unlike most allergic responses, occur quickly, usually within 20 minutes or so after ingestion of a sulfited food.

Sulfites also destroy vitamin B_1 (thiamine), which is why meats and other foods that are known to be major sources of this vitamin are not allowed to contain them. Yet, once again, a lot still do! For instance, many of today's bran cereals (fine thiamine source) contain dried fruits preserved with sulfites. And though soy protein, frozen vegetables, and fruit juices might not be *major* sources of thiamine, they are good ones, especially if consumed daily. But their sulfite content can negate any potentially significant vitamin B_1 contribution to your diet.

27. Protecting Yourself Against Sulfites

If you have allergies, asthma, or suspect that you are sensitive to sulfites, you can protect yourself in several ways:

• Consult a doctor or allergist to confirm that you *are* sulfite-sensitive and ask if you can be desensitized. Most people can. (There is no need to live in fear of unexpected side effects or have to avoid so many nutritious but potentially dangerous foods. See section 28.)

• Read labels and avoid foods with any sulfiting agents.

• Don't trust salad bars. (The food might have been sulfited by the produce supplier before it even reached the restaurant.)

• Avoid dried fruits. (Some asthmatics can have attacks simply from smelling a freshly opened package of dried apricots.)

• Throw away the outside leaves of any lettuce or celery purchased at supermarkets.

• Ask at restaurants if your food contains sulfites. (They might not know or they might not tell you, but it doesn't hurt to ask. If you're still worried, order something not sulfited—broiled chicken, meat, or an omelette without vegetables, for instance.)

• Check your local pharmacy for a new sulfite test strip that is designed to produce a virtually instantaneous red color when touched to a sulfite-containing food. (The darker the red, the more sulfite in the food.)

• Take nutritional supplements that can help minimize allergic and asthmatic reactions. (Highly allergic individuals should, nevertheless, strictly avoid sulfites!) I would suggest:

High-potency multiple vitamin with chelated minerals, A.M. and P.M.

Vitamin B complex, 100 mg., 3 times daily
Pantothenic acid, 100 mg., 3 times daily
Vitamin E (dry form), 200–400 IU, 2–3 times daily
Vitamin C, 500 mg., 2–3 times daily

CAUTION: If you are on tetracycline medication, vitamin C buffered with calcium ascorbate can interfere with the medicine's effectiveness. You can use a sodium ascorbate form of vitamin C with tetracyclines, but *not* if you're on a sodium-restricted diet or are taking steroids. *This regimen is not intended as medical advice. Before starting any supplement program or making dietary changes, check "Cautions" in section 126 and with your physician or a nutritionally oriented doctor. (See section 143.)*

28. Know Your Most Frequently Sulfited Foods

Whether sulfites occur naturally, as they do in wines (without sulfites you'd have a lot of vintage vinegar), or are added later, they're equally dangerous if you have a sulfite sensitivity. Remember, just because a sulfite is not on the label doesn't mean it is not in the product.

MOST FREQUENTLY SULFITED FOODS

Baked Products

Cookies, crackers (even good old grahams), pie and quiche crusts, soft pretzels, waffles, wheat tortillas

Beverages
(Canned, bottled, frozen, regular, and dietetic)

Beer, cider, cocktail mixes, colas, fruit drinks, fruit juices, instant tea, soups, vegetable juices, wine coolers, wines

Candies, Confections, Desserts, and Syrups

Caramels, hard candies (sour balls, etc.), brown sugar, raw beet sugar, powdered beet sugar, white granulated beet sugar, corn sugar, Maraschino cherries, glazed fruits, jellies, jams, corn syrup, maple syrup, pancake syrup, fruit toppings, high fructose corn syrup, shredded coconut, flavored (and unflavored) gelatins, fruit pie fillings

Fish
(Frozen, canned, dried, and fresh)

Clams, crab, dried cod, lobster, scallops, shrimp; also canned seafood soups

Pastas, Grains, and Other Carbohydrates

Spinach pasta, cornstarch, modified food starch, breadings, noodle and rice mixes, potato chips, processed potato salad, hominy

Relishes, Condiments, and Mixes

Horeseradish, pickles, olives, onion relish, salad dressing mixes, wine vinegar, pickled vegetables, sauerkraut, coleslaw, guacamole, gravies (including those that are milk-based), dried soup mixes

Vegetables and Fruits
(Canned, frozen, dried, instant, cut-up fresh)

Mushrooms, grapes, prepared cut fruit or vegetable salads, shredded cabbage, avocado salad, dried fruits, trail mixes, breakfast cereals with dried fruit, dried fruit snacks or dietetic processed fruits

29. Vitamins Can Be Additives, Too

Vitamins are frequently added to foods for other than nutritional reasons and listed as ingredients under their chemical names. Since unfamiliar and unpronounceable ingredients have come to be regarded by health-conscious consumers as dangerous (admittedly, not without some reason), many nutritious products using vitamins as additives are being unnecessarily avoided.

A vitamin by any other name is still a vitamin—even when it's an additive. That doesn't mean vitamins are all risk free for everyone all the time (see "Cautions" in section 126), but I believe their benefit-risk ration as additives beats that of the competition's.

VITAMINS AS ADDITIVES

VITAMIN	POSSIBLE LISTING ON LABELS
A	Vitamin A acetate, Vitamin A palmitate
B_1	Thiamine hydrochloride, thiamine mononitrate
B_2	Riboflavin, riboflavin-5-phosphate, sodium riboflavin phosphate (disodium riboflavin phosphate), lactoflavin
B_5	Pantothenic acid, calcium pantothenate
B_6	Pyridoxine hydrochloride
B_{12}	Cyanocobalamin
B_c	Folacin, folic acid
C	Ascorbic acid, sodium ascorbate

VITAMIN	POSSIBLE LISTING ON LABELS
D	Vitamin D_2 (ergocalciferol); vitamin D_3 (cholecalciferol, 7-dehydrocholesterol)
E	Tocopherols, alpha-tocopherol, alpha-tocopherol acetate
G	Riboflavin (see B_2)
H	Biotin, vitamin B factor
K	Menadione (vitamin K_3), menaquinone (vitamin K_2), phylloquinone (vitamin K_1), phytonadione

30. Any Questions About Chapter 2?

How do scientists know how much of an additive is safe for human consumption when the tests are all done on animals?

They don't. They can only determine what they "consider" safe, based on the level (amount of additive substance) that is found to cause *no* adverse effects in animal feeding experiments. This level is then used to calculate a margin of safety for human consumption, usually a hundred times the safe animal level, establishing the additive's intake in milligrams per kilogram of body weight.

I'm confused. Does a "fortified" product have more or less additives than an "enriched" one?

Your confusion is understandable. Although fortification and enrichment are not the same, there is no legal distinction between them.

Essentially, fortification is adding nutrients to foods that never contained them (imitation fruit drinks, for instance). This means that inexpensive synthetic vitamins and minerals can be added to sugary junk foods to make them appear nutritious so they can sell for more.

Enrichment, on the other hand, is replacing nutrients in foods that once contained them. These nutrients are lost as a result of heat, storage, and so forth. Foods are enriched to the levels found in the natural product before processing.

Whether an enriched food has more additives than a fortified one depends on the product. My feeling, though, is to be wary of fortified products, since (with a few exceptions) most are just boosting their nutrient content to sell more of a naturally non-nutritious food for more money.

Could you please tell me what HVP is and if it's safe? And I would also like to know what it's doing in onion soup.

Classified as an additive, HVP (hydrolyzed vegetable protein), sometimes called HPP (hydrolyzed plant protein), is frequently listed on labels as hydrolyzed cereal solids.

It's obtained through a chemical splitting of soybean and peanut meals, or crude protein from already wet milled wheat, corn, or other grain by water processing (hydrolysis). I'd say that it's not harmful as long as people know that it has a high salt content and are aware of the dangers of eating too much salt. (See section 93.)

Since its prime use is as a flavor enhancer, my guess is that's what it's doing in your onion soup. (It is frequently in soup mixes, gravies, and chili to provide a meaty flavor.)

Is the hydrolyzed casein in my liquid diet meals a nutrient or a whole food?

It's a manufactured additive, used as a nutritional supplement and an amino acid source in infant formulas, that is made from the principal protein in milk (casein). Because it is enzymatically hydrolyzed, it contains substantial amounts of glutamic acid, an amino acid formed by hydrolysis that has been found to affect the central nervous system and the brain of infants, and produce a lethal imbalance of amino acids when comsumed as a total "liquid protein diet." Its use in infant formulas is still being studied, as well it should. When hydrolyzed casein is consumed exclusively, or as the main part of an unsupplemented diet, it can cause death.

Liquid protein diets, which are composed primarily of hydrolyzed casein, are unsafe without adequate and balanced supplementation. They keep the body from using its own organs and muscles to meet protein needs. These diets were designed to promote large weight losses quickly; unfortunately, our national flirtation with anorexia has brought them fast popularity and sent more than one dieter to the grave. Without medical supervision, I would not advise you to drink them as a replacement for more than one meal daily. In fact, I'd recommend that you steer clear of them completely.

3
IS THIS ANY WAY TO START A DAY?

31. The Meal Most Likely to
Breakfast is the meal most likely to...

- Affect learning ability and reaction time.
- Influence vitality and fitness.
- Be rushed, unplanned, eaten on the run, and missed.

It is also the most important meal of the day—and the most nutritionally abused.

32. Breakfasts That DON'T Make Your Day
Breakfast comes after the longest period of time that your body has been without food. If your internal systems are inadequately or improperly replenished, they are going to let you down. You can't expect high performance running on empty.

Most people know this and feel that any breakfast is better than none. But you won't get high performance using the wrong fuel either. Obviously, this is not as well known, as evidenced by the more than six million people who drink Coca-Cola for breakfast and the popularity of the following morning meals:

THE OFFICE QUICKIE

A doughnut or pastry grabbed on the run and washed down with coffee. Regarded as a "something to hold you until lunch"

44

meal, its subversive qualities, such as diminishing alertness throughout the morning and increasing midday fatigue, are not widely known— but they are experienced by millions daily.

Trade-off Suggestions: Instead of a high-fat, high-sugar pastry, try a bagel. Bagels are low in fat, contain more protein than two slices of bread (and about the same amount of calories), and are now available with more fiber in whole-grain varieties. Instead of spreading it with cream cheese (which would defeat the trade-off since cream cheese has more than 2 teaspoons of fat per ounce), try apple butter, or a really thin slice of Swiss or Cheddar cheese topped with a tomato.

Low-fat cottage cheese mixed with either chopped scallions or fruit-flavored yogurt works well, too. But if you really feel that a bagel is not a bagel without cream cheese, use a *thin* layer of *light* cream cheese. You'll get all the flavor, only half the fat, and be a whole lot healthier for it.

CAUTION: Bagels are made with high-gluten flour and are contraindicated for anyone with celiac disease.

FROZEN BREAKFAST SANDWICHES

Like Egg McMuffins and Croissan 'wiches, these microwavable breakfasts on buns are time-saving time bombs loaded with sodium and fat. One Great Starts Sausage Biscuit, for example, contains a whopping 1,565 mg. of sodium (no more than 1,100 to 3,300 mg. of sodium should be consumed *in a day*) and 52 percent of its hefty 430 calories come from fat. Considering that no more than 20 percent of a healthful daily diet's calories should be derived from fat, that is a risky way to start any day—particularly since products of this type also contain colorings and additives (some potentially carcinogenic) that can cause numerous unpleasant reactions in susceptible individuals (see section 24).

Trade-off Suggestions: If you like the convenience of a hot breakfast on a muffin, but don't want all the sodium, fat, and additives that come with it, make your own. Spread it with peanut butter, add a slice of cheese, microwave on high for about 40 seconds (or put in a toaster oven until the cheese melts), and you'll save a lot more than time. For variation, try a thin slice of cheese and a slice of nitrite-free bacon or ham; or low-fat cottage cheese, sprinkled with cinnamon, on a raisin muffin.

NO-FUSS FRENCH TOAST, WAFFLES, AND PANCAKES

Now that they are microwavable, these classic breakfast treats are being served with increasing frequency in busy households, subjecting more unwary people, more often, to an unhealthy on-slaught of excessive salt, sugar, potentially carcinogenic preserva-tives and coal tar–based dyes. (And that's not counting what is in whatever syrups, jellies, or jams might be used as toppings!) Though convenient and tasty, these no-fuss processed breakfasts can raise blood pressure, lower spirits, and, if eaten on a regular basis, become significant contributing factors to serious ailments.

Trade-off Suggestions: If you're going to eat these breakfasts despite their nutritional negatives, read labels before buying. Com-pare the ingredients of different brands, then select whichever has the lowest amount of saturated fat and the highest amount of fiber. Choose products made with bran and whole wheat flour over those that are not.

FAST, FULL-COURSE FIRST MEALS

There is nothing like a good, nutritious breakfast—and the microwavable morning entrees now being marketed are nothing like good, nutritious breakfasts. Whether the meals sound down-home familiar (Great Starts Scrambled Eggs & Sausage with Hashed Brown Potatoes, for instance) or gourmet exotic (Cafe Classics Eggs Enchilada), the sodium and fat levels are equally and appallingly high. Cholesterol watchers, watch out! What these beat-the-clock breakfasts save you in time, you pay for in health. They contain between 360 and 500 mg. of cholesterol—250 to 300 mg. more than recommended for a whole day. Additionally, all have fewer nutrients and more additives than they should, and harbor numerous poten-tial catalysts for adverse reactions in susceptible individuals (see section 24).

Trade-off Suggestions: If you want scrambled eggs and sausage, you're better off buying the sausage separately (choosing the brand with the least amount of harmful additives) and scrambling your own preservative-free eggs. Also, heating up last night's leftovers can make a better full-course breakfast than you'll get in a box.

33. Getting the Juice on the Juice

Frozen, canned, cartoned, bottled, or fresh orange juice is a real eye-opener—in ways that can make you think before you drink.

JUICY EYE-OPENERS

• Orange juice is the most popular natural source of vitamin C, but not the best. (An 8-ounce cup of orange juice has approximately 124 mg. of vitamin C; an 8-ounce cup of cooked broccoli contains 140 mg.

• The vitamin C content of all oranges is not the same. (Different varieties contain different amounts, and these amounts increase or decrease depending on how early or late in their growing season the oranges are picked. Generally, the later they are picked, the lower their vitamin C content.)

• The vitamin C content of reconstituted frozen orange juice can vary from brand to brand by as much as 100 percent. (Wide variations in vitamin C content can also occur within a single brand.)

• All oranges are not orange. (Florida oranges are frequently green when they're ripe and dyed orange to please consumers.)

• The nutritional value of orange juice, fresh or processed, is highly overrated. (Except for its vitamin C and potassium, orange juice provides you with little more than carbohydrates in the form of the natural sugars sucrose, fructose, and glucose.)

• Fresh squeezed or unsweetened orange juice is not a low-calorie drink. (It's actually higher in calories than many soft drinks.)

• A lot of expensive "fresh-squeezed" juice sold in cartons comes from last year's oranges. (As long as the oranges were fresh when they were squeezed, and the juice was not concentrated before it was frozen for storage, the manufacturer can blend last year's juice with current squeezings—squeezing out extra profits.)

• Canned and bottled juices (those that are stored and sold

unrefrigerated) have about the same amount of vitamin C as frozen concentrates made from the same type of oranges being canned at a particular time, but their flavor tends to deteriorate. They also tend to have greater amounts of insect debris than other forms of orange juice. (Their only real advantage is that they can be stored without refrigeration. For ready-to-pour convenience, you're better off with reconstituted juice sold in cartons, which costs, ounce for ounce, about the same—with some store-label brand exceptions—and tastes better.)

　• The FDA limits on amounts of "natural and unavoidable" debris in citrus juices are unappetizingly high, they don't cover all kinds of debris, and USDA inspection does not guarantee exceptional cleanliness. (I'm not saying that allowable insect debris is a health hazard, but unless you're a bird, frog, or other arthropodan eater by choice, it's certainly no taste turn-on either.)

34. Know Your Oranges

If you are going to squeeze your own juice, you're not likely to be helped in your selection by federal grade standards. Aside from the use of several grading systems (which is confusing when you discover that an orange grade "No. 1" is better than one graded "No. 1 Bright" as long as it is not from Florida, where that grade is reversed), oranges are graded primarily on appearance, shape, and color, which is not necessarily relevant to nutritional value or taste.

DOs & DON'Ts FOR PICKING A GOOD JUICY ORANGE

DON'T buy any with soft spots, cuts, punctures, or spongy skin.
DO select the firmest and heaviest ones over the lightweights.
DON'T judge by color. (Many undyed oranges are greenish when ripest, and Florida and Texas oranges speckled with brown or black flecks are often thin-skinned and top-quality.)
DO choose those with smooth, fresh-looking skin.
DON'T select by name unless you know that variety's growing season. (Generally, the later in its season, the less the orange's vitamin C content.)

DO keep in mind that a medium-sized orange (approximately 6 ounces) will provide about 2 to 2½ ounces of juice. (The average small breakfast portion served is 3½ ounces.)

GOOD NAMES, SEASONS, AND ''Cs'' TO REMEMBER

VARIETY	SEASON	APPROXIMATE VITAMIN C IN 3½ OUNCES OF JUICE
Valencia (CA)	April–October	60 mg.–42 mg.
Valencia (FL)	Late March–June	45 mg.–22 mg.
Temple (FL)	Early January–early March	51 mg.
Hamlin (FL)	Early October–December	55 mg.–36 mg.
Pineapple (FL)	December–February	60 mg.–50 mg.
Parson Brown (FL)	Early November–January	52 mg.–47 mg.

35. Hold the Bacon, Please!

There is nothing bad about bacon that not eating it won't cure. It's high in saturated fat and high in sodium. It contains nitrite, an additive that can react with natural chemicals in our foods and bodies to form nitrosamines, potent cancer-causing substances. And to heighten the health risks, it is an inconsistent product at best.

> If you bring home the bacon, don't fry it.

A pig's age, sex, and diet affect how it accumulates fat. This causes significant variations in the pork bellies manufacturers buy for use as bacon. Consequently, taste, as well as protein, fat, sodium, and so forth, can vary not only from brand to brand but from package to package!

But more than quality and uniformity are involved. Even though there are legal limits to the amount of nitrites allowed, and specified vitamin C compounds that must be added to retard nitrosamine formation during processing, the product's inconsistency precludes assurance that every package of bacon has nitrosamine levels within USDA standards. In other words, the chances of your bacon having more nitrosamines than it should are more than likely. Add to that the fact that no level of nitrosamine is "safe," and you have to concede that bringing home the bacon can be a health-risky business.

If you are a confirmed bacon lover, expecting you to give up your beloved morning breakfast treat because of its potential health hazard is as realistic as getting confirmed smokers to quit. But you can at least minimize the risks.

CUTTING BACK ON BACON RISKS

• Select bacon with the most meat and least fat. (Nitrosamine levels are higher in fat.)

• Don't use bacon grease for cooking. (It contains nearly four times the nitrosamines as the bacon!)

• Instead of frying, cook bacon on paper towels in a microwave. (This produces less nitrosamines.) If you don't have a microwave, broil or oven-fry the bacon at a fairly low temperature. It will take longer, but fewer nitrosamines will be produced.

• Always cook bacon in a well-ventilated area. (Some nitrosamines can vaporize during cooking, and they are easily inhaled.) It's wise to discourage young children in particular from sniffing those cooking aromas.

• Use nitrite-free bacon. (It's not as tasty, but it's not as dangerous either.)

• Don't be fooled into thinking that baconlike products (Sizzlean, Tastystrips, etc.) are safer than the real thing. They use sodium nitrite for their cured taste and pink/red color, too.

• Eat bacon as an occasional treat. (Making it frequent or everyday fare is just asking for trouble.)

MY SUGGESTION: If you do indulge in bacon, be sure you're ingesting enough vitamins C, A, D, and E to help counteract the nitrites. (For best natural sources, see section 128.) I'd also recommend the following daily supplement regimen:

• One high-potency multiple vitamin with chelated minerals (time release preferred), taken with breakfast or dinner

- Vitamin C, 500–1,000 mg., 1–3 times daily
- Vitamin E (dry form), 200–400 IU, 1–2 times daily

36. Do Eggs Have a Sunny Side?

The American Heart Association doesn't seem to think so; it still feels that more than three egg yolks a week can be hazardous. On the other hand, most nutritionists, members of the American Medical Association, and the National Research Council feel otherwise.

There is no controversy about the connection between cholesterol and heart disease. Innumerable studies have proven that your risk of heart attack increases when cholesterol levels in the blood become abnormally high. But whether or not eating eggs elevates serum cholesterol and triglycerides (blood fats) is another matter—one with enough cons and pros to fill a penitentiary.

UNSCRAMBLING THE FACTS

- Lipoproteins are factors in our blood which transport cholesterol, and cholesterol behaves differently depending on the protein to which it is bound.
- Very low-density lipoproteins (VLDL) have been found to bear a correlation to heart disease.
- High-density lipoproteins (HDL), which are composed principally of lecithin whose detergent action breaks up cholesterol so that it is transported through the blood without clogging arteries, have been found to help prevent heart disease.
- Eggs not only have the most perfect protein components of any food, but they also contain lecithin—and they *raise* HDL levels!

ON THE DOWN SIDE	ON THE SUNNY SIDE
Some people suffer from a condition known as *Type IV lipidemia,* a hereditary inability to metabolize cholesterol. For them, eggs (despite their lecithin content) could still raise serum cholesterol levels.	Most people don't have this condition.

ON THE DOWN SIDE	ON THE SUNNY SIDE
Many people, particularly children, are allergic to eggs.	Usually the egg whites (primarily albumen), not the yolks, cause the allergic reactions.
Eggs are often fried in butter, bacon grease, and other saturated fats that can heighten the risk of heart disease and other ailments.	They can be fried without saturated fats in non-stick pans, or pans lightly greased with unsaturated oil.
They are easy to consume in excess, putting a strain on the kidneys to excrete the nitrogenous products of protein metabolism—which can also lead to a loss of calcium.	They're just as easy to consume in moderation, and better for you that way.

NOTE: If you're allergic to eggs, you might also react adversely to products containing the additive *lactalbumin phosphate*. Check labels. It's frequently used in imitation dairy products, diet supplements, baked goods, frostings, breakfast cereals, fruit drinks, and sweet sauces, among others.

37. Cold Starters

Ready-to-eat cereals are plentiful, popular, and puffed up with nutrition claims. If they aren't boasting "less sugar" or "high fiber," it's "added nutrients" or "100% natural ingredients"—and it's all just more misleading advertising baloney. Unfortunately, millions are swallowing it by the bowlful every morning.

THE NAME GAME

Names of products are changed to make them appear more wholesome. For example, Post's Super Sugar Crisp is now Super Golden Crisp, though its 3.5 teaspoons of sugar per serving are still the same. Kellogg's Sugar Frosted Flakes has slimmed down to Frosted Flakes, but the 2.8 teaspoons of sugar in its one-ounce servings are still the same. And despite Sugar Smacks being transformed to Honey Smacks, most of the cereal's sweetness still comes from sugar.

THE HIDE-THE-SUGAR GAME

Now that people are more aware of the dangers of too much sugar (see section 63), manufacturers are trying to disguise its presence in their product by saying it is flavored with naturally sweet fruit juice. Nabisco 100% Bran, for instance, is flavored with "two naturally sweet fruit juices" and contains more sugar than either. And most of Kellogg's OJ's sweetness—despite the ½ teaspoon of orange concentrate per serving—comes from sugar.

THE HIDE-THE-SALT GAME

Simply because a cereal is low in sugar doesn't mean it is necessarily healthier for you. For example, whole wheat Wheaties, called "the breakfast of champions," is low in sugar but contains 370 mg. of sodium per ounce—not what I consider a winning way to start the day. In fact, many ready-to-eat cereals have been riding high on their low-sugar content while insidiously supplying more sodium per ounce than potato chips! A one-ounce portion of Wise Potato Chips has approximately 190 mg. of salt; a one-ounce portion of Cheerios has 290 mg., Kix has 315 mg., Total and Kellogg's Corn Flakes have 280 mg. Children brought up on salty foods are more likely to become hooked on them in later life. And too much salt is just as much a health hazard as too much sugar (see section 93).

THE PRESWEETENED MYTH GAME

Manufacturers claim that the reason they presweeten cereals— frequently to sugary levels of 3½ teaspoons per ounce—is to prevent consumers, particularly children, from adding too much sugar on their own. Now, really! How much more could they add? At this point, most presweetened cereals are little more than fortified candy. They might say they provide ten or more essential vitamins and minerals, but that doesn't mean you're getting them. Additionally, refined sugars (which presweetened cereals contain) deplete the body of B-complex vitamins, which are necessary for the proper assimilation of other vitamins and minerals.

Despite labels stating how many grams of sugar an ounce contains, few people realize what this figure converts to in teaspoons. An ounce of cereal is not a large portion, but it is considered a serving. And a single serving of a cereal like Cap'n Crunch, for instance, with half a cup of milk, contains 18 g. of sugar—*nearly 4 teaspoons!*

THE FIBER-BRAN-BANDWAGON GAME

With substantial evidence that fiber can protect us from ailments ranging from constipation to cancer, manufacturers have jumped on the fiber-bran bandwagon with cereals galore. But all fiber is not the same (see section 101), and some of the most popular high-fiber cereals have enough sodium, sugar, and additives to counteract their potential benefits for many individuals. Hypertensives, diabetics, asthmatics, and anyone with gastrointestinal problems, for instance, should be aware that Kellogg's Fruitful Bran's 4 g. of dietary fiber comes with 230 mg. of sodium, 11 g. of sugar, sulfur dioxide (see section 26), and sorbitol (see section 66), which may alter the absorption of some drugs, making them less effective or more toxic.

General Mills' Fiber One offers 12 g. of dietary fiber, but is accompanied by 220 mg. of sodium and contains aspartame (see section 67), which can adversely affect individuals with phenylketonuria (PKU), elevate blood pressure, is contraindicated for anyone taking MAO inhibitors, and is not recommended for epileptics or pregnant women.

Post's Fruit & Fibre, which has 4 g. of dietary fiber, is also not the best breakfast bet for asthmatics, allergic individuals, and hypertensives, since it contains sulfur dioxide, artificial flavors, *and* BHA.

Kellogg's Cracklin' Oat Bran, cashing in on the research that has shown the health benefits of soluble fiber (see section 101), contains more sugar than diabetics should have and four or more times as much fat as other cereals, with the exception of commercial granolas.

Despite drawbacks, most dry high-fiber cereals have more nutrition benefits than other ready-to-eat cereals. But in order to reap these benefits, disregard advertising hype, read labels carefully, and select cereals that, for you, have the least amount of potentially harmful ingredients.

Trade-off Suggestions for Cold Cereals: Preservative-free wheat flake and millet flake dry cereals. (Difficult to find in supermarkets, but worth a trip to your local natural food store.)

Unsweetened wheat germ, toasted or raw. (Toasted is tastier, but raw has more vitamins. To get the best of both, buy the wheat germ raw and toast it at home over a low flame in a dry pan. Refrigerate the unused portion in a tightly sealed jar.)

Homemade granola. (By making it without coconut, which contains a lot of saturated fat, and going easy on the oil and sweeteners, you can enjoy its nutritious benefits without compromising your health.) The following recipe makes about a pound and is as simple as it is delicious.

GREAT GRANOLA

Heat 2 tbsp. honey, 2 tbsp. sunflower or sesame seed oil, and ⅛ tsp. vanilla. Pour this over a mixture of 1½ cups oats; ¼ cup wheat germ; ¾ cup chopped peanuts, almonds, and sesame, pumpkin, and sunflower seeds; and ¼ cup currants or raisins. Spread on shallow, flat pan and bake in a 325° F. oven for 10 minutes, stir to prevent sticking, then continue baking for another 10 minutes, or until toasty brown.

(To further minimize fat intake, serve with low-fat yogurt or applesauce.)

38. What's Hot and What's Not

Refinement might be socially commendable in people, but it is nutritionally reprehensible in cereals. In fact, the more refined grains are, the more reason for you to have less to do with them.

Whether a cereal has been dutifully enriched with synthetic replacements for lost nutrients or summarily degerminated (stripped of all but the kernel's starchy endosperm, then minimally reimbursed with synthetic substitutes), it is still refined—and capable of shortchanging you of important vitamins and minerals.

Many of these cereals are seductively appealing because they are quick-cooking, "instant" types. All the more reason for scrutinizing their labels and avoiding those that contain disodium phosphate, an additive suspected of causing teeth and bone deterioration and kidney problems.

NOT SO HOT CEREALS

Cream of wheat, cream of rice, farina, and hominy, which for years have been accepted as top-notch, high-nutrition hot breakfasts, are not, I'm sorry to say, the cream of the crop. All of them are degerminated—processed for creaminess by eliminating all grain germ and bran.

Trade-off Suggestion: Whole-grain, stone-ground yellow cornmeal. It's as creamy as any of the cereals, but is not degerminated.

THE HOT ONES

Oatmeal, with no sugar or salt, is an old-fashioned wholesome breakfast with a new plus going for it—oat bran, a soluble fiber that's been shown to help diabetics lower insulin requirements and aid in fighting heart disease by reducing serum cholesterol levels in low-fat diets.

Several oat bran cereals are now on the market. The best are those in which rolled oats, oat bran, or oat bran and another whole grain (wheat bran, wheat germ, etc.) are the only ingredients. The worst are highly processed (usually the "instant" type), and unhealthily endowed with natural and/or artificial sweeteners, sulfur dioxide, BHA, and a high sodium content. Such ingredients can negate the beneficial effects of oat bran, and pose health risks for hypertensives and diabetics. (See section 101 for the differences between soluble and insoluble fiber.)

Cereals made with unrefined wheat, Wheatena for example, are old standbys with a lot of contemporary nutritional merit (see section 114 for grains that do and don't make the grade), providing you don't subvert this by slathering them with sugar, butter, and salt. Admittedly, plain gran cereals *sans* such flavorings are not turn-ons for modern taste buds, but these are healthier alternatives. I'm not going to tell you that these will impart the same flavor, because they won't. But they won't set you up for heart disease, diabetes, or arteriosclerosis, either—and, given a chance, they'll provide you not only with a way to enjoy more nutritious, and addititve-free, foods more often, but, in many cases, to get extra vitamins and minerals as well.

INSTEAD OF	TRY FLAVORING WITH . . .
Refined sugar	Fruit juice, honey, raisins, fresh fruits (apricots, peaches, seedless grapes, strawberries), a dash of pure maple syrup or blackstrap molasses. (If you like blueberries, coat a handful with honey and then add them to your cereal for a fiber bonus and a taste treat.) **CAUTION:** If you are taking an anticoagulant (blood thinner), don't use blackstrap molasses. It's high in vitamin K and can reverse the effect of your medication.
1 tablespoon butter	1 tablespoon whipped margarine (has no cholesterol and only 2.1 g. of saturated fat, as opposed to butter's 33 mg. of cholesterol and 6.3 g. saturated fat), or peanut butter (no cholesterol and only 1.5 g. saturated fat).
Salt	Cinnamon or nutmeg
Whole milk	Low-fat or skim milk, or buttermilk; plain low fat yogurt (add your own fresh fruit)

39. Breads You Might Not Propose to Toast

Practically all breads you find in today's supermarkets have been processed and depleted of nutrients that are then replaced through *enrichment*—a euphemism if there ever was one. The standard of enrichment for white flour is replacing twenty-two natural nutrients with three B vitamins, vitamin D, calcium, and iron salts. That's not what I'd call enrichment, particularly since there is no guarantee that your body can utilize all, or any, of those added nutrients.

WHITE BREAD

Regrettably, America's favorite, white bread, is made from highly processed wheat flour that has been milled and bleached, and therefore depleted of numerous nutrients that enrichment cannot replace. Ironically, this has a redeeming feature. The processing causes the eradication of phytic acid, a chemical found in numerous whole grains that can prevent the body from using many minerals contained in flour. On the other hand, this is a dubious plus: Phytic acid has been found to help in the prevention of colon cancer. Weighing the pluses and minuses, the minuses have it.

• White bread contains mono- and diglycerides to maintain "softness." Though present in small amounts, these glycerides can insidiously increase saturated fat intakes because they are unknowingly being ingested regularly and frequently.
• Its formula is standardized by the Code of Federal Regulations and therefore the bread may contain more than a hundred food and chemical additives that need not be listed on the label!
• Even when made with unbleached flour, it is still lacking the two main constituents of the whole wheat kernel: bran (the outermost, vitamin B–rich fiber layer) and germ (the sprouting section that contains polyunsaturated fats, vitamin E, and other important nutrients).
• It can claim "no preservatives" and still contain dough conditioners, such as potassium bromate (which has been known to cause central nervous system disorders and kidney problems) and sodium stearoyl lactylate, as well as chemical yeast nutrients such as calcium and ammonium sulfate (the former frequently used in wall plaster and the latter in fireproofing fabrics), among others.

Minimize the Negatives:

• If you are going to buy white bread, at least make sure that it is enriched.

• Choose products with the lowest sodium and fat, the most added nutrients, and no BHA.

• Buy thin-sliced, instead of regular, products.

• Choose breads made with unbleached flour over those made with white flour (often listed as "flour") or wheat flour, which is the same as white flour.

• Avoid commercial packaged breads with added calcium or sodium propionate (a bread made with quality ingredients under proper conditions doesn't need these added fresheners).

• Cover your lost nutrient bases with a daily high-potency multiple vitamin and mineral supplement that has at least 50 mg. of vitamins B_1, B_2, and B_6, and zinc.

Trade-off Suggestions: Hard-crusted, enriched Italian or French breads, which are soft and white inside, generally use unbleached flour and contain no sugar or animal fat.

Pita breads, which are great for sandwiches, contain no sugar or shortening at all.

DARK BREADS
(Whole wheat, rye, oatmeal, pumpernickel, etc.)

Breads made from unrefined flour containing the entire bran, germ, and endosperm of grains are matchless sources of natural, life-sustaining nutrients. Unfortunately, most people never get to eat them. Modern milling processes and corporate profit quests have made their manufacture economically undesirable, and consumer gullibility has made it unnecessary.

Manufacturers have discovered that just about any brown bread packaged with words such as "natural" or "fiber-rich" (particularly in old-fashioned lettering) can be passed off as nutritious. But until consumers wise up, the proverbial "staff of life" will continue to be just another flimsy stick. Just because a bread is dark does not necessarily mean that it's nutritious, or that it's the right bread for you.

• Many brown breads have little if any whole grains and are essentially white breads that have been colored with molasses. (Appearances, like labels, can be and often are deceiving.)
• Dark breads are not inherently beneficial for all people. Breads made with whole wheat, rye, oats, and barley can worsen the health of individuals with celiac disease.
• Breads labeled "natural wheat" or "stone ground" may not be whole wheat products. Unless "whole wheat" is listed as the *first* ingredient, the bread isn't.
• Wheat flour is *not* the same as whole wheat flour. Actually, it is so far from it that it's virtually the same as bleached white flour—low in nutrients and full of chemicals.
• Many whole-grain breads, rich as they are in B vitamins, also contain preservatives that can deplete them.
• Some whole-grain breads use caramel color, which, despite its natural source, is a suspected carcinogen, and is under investigation for possible mutagenic properties.

Minimize the Negatives:

• Avoid breads made with hydrogenated shortening, dough conditioners, yeast nutrients, emulsifiers, or fresheners.
• Choose breads made with whole wheat flour over others.
• Select loaves made with vegetable oil and butter over those made with shortening. (Shortening is usually animal fat or partially saturated vegetable fat and generally contains emulsifiers and other preservatives.)

40. Choosing Your Morning Bread Spreads

Whether it's a bagel, muffin, or just plain toast, what you spread on it for flavor daily can influence your well-being for life. Since so many breakfast spreads are high in saturated fats, cholesterol, salt, sugar, and additives—and are eaten so frequently—discovering which ones are safest and healthiest for you is essential.

BUTTER

Unadulterated Facts:

• The best butter is made from sweet cream and graded "U.S. Grade AA."

• One tablespoon of ordinary (not "sweet" or "unsalted") butter contains 102 calories, 6.3 g. saturated fat, 4.1 g. unsaturated fat, 35 mg. cholesterol, and 140 mg. sodium.

• Salt helps preserve butter, but is often used to cover up off-flavors and staleness in inferior brands.

• Poor-quality butter (made from soured milk or cream with a lot of added salt to inhibit mold) often has an added alkaline salt to neutralize its salty taste.

• Virtually all commercial butters contain natural or artificial coloring, but need not state this on the label.

• Rancid butter can destroy fat-soluble vitamins in your body. (If it smells stale or looks odd, return it or throw it out.)

COMMENTS AND CAUTIONS: Use sweet not salted butter (you don't need extra sodium *and* saturated fat). I also advise using softened or whipped butter because it spreads more easily and you'll use less. Another way to minimize your intake of saturated fat is to blend butter with a quality margarine. You'll still have the butter flavor, but less cholesterol. (Gradually increasing the ratio of margarine to butter might help you make the switch.)

MARGARINE

Unadulterated Facts:

• Some margarines are made from animal fat (making them just as saturated as butter) or a combination of animal and vegetable fat (making them cheaper than butter but not healthier).

• One tablespoon of margarine contains 102 calories (68 if whipped), 2.1 g. saturated fat (1.4 g. if whipped), 9 g. unsaturated fat (6 g. if whipped), 140 mg. of salt (93 mg. if whipped), and no cholesterol.

• Most margarines are made primarily from vegetable fat and oils that contain varying amounts of unsaturated fats. But when these are hydrogenated, or partially hydrogenated (to obtain the consistency of butter that is desired for marketing), many wind up being almost as saturated as butter.

• With the exception of cottonseed oil (contained in virtually all "pure vegetable oils"), which has been exposed to more than a healthy share of chemical pesticides because cotton is not considered a food crop, the type of oil used is less important than how much it has been hydrogenated or hardened.

• *Liquid* vegetable oils low in saturated fats and high in polyunsaturates are best, provided they are listed as the products' *first* ingredient. Tops in polyunsaturates are safflower oil (10 g. per tablespoon), sunflower oil (8.9 g. per tablespoon), soybean oil (8.1 g. per tablespoon), and corn oil (7.8 g. per tablespoon).

• If a label's first ingredient listing is any oil that has been partially hydrogenated or hardened, saturated fat predominates in the product.

• As a general rule, the softer the margarine, the less saturated it is.

COMMENTS AND CAUTIONS: All margarines contain additives, so read labels and avoid products containing any that might be potentially harmful to you (see sections 22 and 24). I'd suggest bypassing any containing EDTA, particularly if you are pregnant or on anticoagulant medication. If you are allergic to milk, Diet Mazola has no milk products and Mother's Sweet Unsalted Margarine has neither milk nor animal products. Avoid any margarines made with coconut or palm oil, which are more saturated than animal fat.

SWEET SPREADS
(Jellies, jams, honey, fruit butters)

Unadulterated Facts:

• Most commercial jams and jellies are not made from fresh fruit. They contain canned, frozen, or strained extracts of frozen fruits.

• These products, with few exceptions, are more than half sugar (only 45 percent is fruit or fruit juice), strictly refined, and sometimes combined with corn syrup. Honey is more expensive and rarely used, yet is the only sweetener that has to be listed on the label.

• Most fruit spreads contain benzoic acid or sodium benzoate (see section 22), artificial colors, flavors, and other additives. But because all ingredients are not required to be listed, many that could be of concern remain unknown.

• Jellies contain approximately 50 calories per tablespoon; jams and preserves approximately 55 calories; apple butter about 33 calories; honey has 64.

• Honey has more fructose than glucose and contains small quantities of minerals, as well as traces of B-complex vitamins and vitamins C, D, and E.

• Because honey is almost twice as sweet as cane or beet sugars, less of it is needed to achieve the same sweetness.

• Some manufacturers will add sugar syrup to their honey because it's cheaper and lightens the honey's color and flavor. (Be suspicious of inexpensive brands that are unusually thin when poured.)

• Some honeys may contain traces of penicillin and sulfite (creating danger for those who are sensitive), as well as cancer-causing substances that the bees extract from the flowers they feed on.

COMMENTS AND CAUTIONS: Sugar in any form poses serious health risks (see section 63) because we eat too much of it—more than 125 pounds per person a year! But if you are determined to have a sweet spread for your morning bread, I'd recommend honey over jam or jelly—although *not* for infants under one year. (It may contain botulinum spores that their systems can't handle.) Because honey is sweeter, a little can provide a lot of flavor—without potentially harmful preservatives or vitamin-depleting refined sugars. Honey labeled "granulated," "creamed," or "spun" is best for spreading. (For more on honey, see section 66.)

Commercial jams and jellies have a lot of sugary negatives, but I don't advise replacing them with their artificially sweetened clones. These contain more potentially harmful additives, many of which don't have to be—and therefore, naturally aren't—listed on the label. You're better off using fruit butter as a spread, even more so if you make it yourself. There is nothing more to it than tossing diced apples, peels and all, into a pot, adding just enough water to prevent sticking, and simmering over a low flame for about an hour and a half, or until the pulp becomes dark and nicely thickened. An equally wholesome and quicker alternative is instant jam: Just mash some fresh berries with a little honey and you have your spread.

CHEESY SPREADABLES
(Pasteurized processed cheese spreads and cream cheese)

Unadulterated Facts:

• With every ounce of pasteurized processed cheese spreads (ground and blended combinations of one or more natural cheeses), you get approximately 4 g. of saturated fat, 16 mg. of cholesterol, 81 calories, and 381 mg. of sodium. But, wait! That's not all. You also get an assortment of artificial colors and flavorings, stabilizers, optional acids, and a combination of more than one dozen different chemicals that you won't find listed on any cheese spread label anywhere.

• One redeeming feature of these spreads (the only one) is that 2 tablespoons, approximately one ounce, contain more calcium (158 mg.) than an entire cup of cottage cheese. But there are better calcium sources (see section 128), and certainly healthier ones.

• Cream cheese, made from fresh, dry, or concentrated milk and water, has a fat content in excess of 37 percent by weight. Whipped, it has approximately one-third less fat per tablespoon (but that's not by weight). In either form, that is a lot of fat.

• An ounce of cream cheese contains 105 calories, 5.8 g. of saturated fat, 3.6 g. of unsaturated fat, 31 mg. of cholesterol, and 70 mg. of sodium.

• Cream cheese is a poor source of protein and calcium.

• Many brands contain propylene glycol alginate (see section 22) and other additives that may pose potential health risks for you. Check labels carefully.

COMMENTS AND CAUTIONS: If you feel that a breakfast bagel without cream cheese is unthinkable, try using Neufchatel cheese. It tastes very much like cream cheese, but has a slightly lower fat content. (Every little dietary subtraction helps.) Personally, I'd recommend trying to reeducate your taste buds. Low-fat cottage cheese is very spreadable and good for you. It can be sprinkled with chives for added zip. (Pot cheese, which is made without salt or additives, is similar but drier.) You might also want to try yogurt cheese, which is low in fat and wholesome on many levels. Be forewarned, though, that this cheese is tart. Then again, once you develop a taste for it, you're likely never to want cream cheese again.

As for using a pasteurized processed cheese spread, my advice is, don't. You are better off melting a thin slice of white Cheddar, which will give you more protein, less sodium, and spare your body from having to cope with a barrage of chemicals the first thing in the morning.

41. Any Questions About Chapter 3?

Should I still be taking a multiple vitamin-mineral supplement if I'm eating a cereal that supplies 100 percent of my daily U.S. RDA requirements?

In my opinion, you have all the more reason to. U.S. RDAs, as explained in section 8, are formulated for labeling purposes and intended only as general recommendations for preventing deficiencies of nineteen essential nutrients. But there are far more than nineteen essential nutrients, even though requirements for them have not yet been established, and everyone's nutrient needs are not the same. And just because a cereal is fortified doesn't mean it's healthful. Kellogg's Most meets 100 percent of the U.S. RDA for eleven vitamins and minerals, but it also contains 2 teaspoons of sugar in every ¾ cup serving, and has been processed with additives that can negate your utilization of many of the added nutrients.

No one food or supplement should be used to supply 100 percent of your need for any nutrient. Variety is more than the spice of life, it's the sustenance of it. But because our foods have been so highly processed and our environment is so filled with pollutants, I feel that taking a daily multiple-vitamin mineral supplement, unless medically contraindicated, is most advisable. As far as vitamin overdosing is concerned, you can safely consume several times the amount of vitamins in any cereal. Most adults would have to consume over 100,000 IU of vitamin A and 25,000 IU of vitamin D daily over an extended period of time to produce toxic effects.

My children never have time for breakfast, so I've been giving them Carnation Instant Breakfast milk shakes. Are these good for them?

The milk is, but I can't say the same for the packaged mix. Not only does it add an extra 135 mg. of sodium to their daily intake, along with artificial flavors, but—most significant—it contains carrageenan, which can interfere with the body's immunological warning system and should be avoided, particularly during illness. Blending your own shakes for them would be just as quick and much healthier. My teenaged daughter Alanna loves this one. (It's great for her skin, too.)

BANANA BONANZA

6 oz. nonfat milk
1 tbsp. nutritional yeast powder (lots of B vitamins)
1 tbsp. acidophilus liquid (promotes friendly bacteria)
1 tbsp. granulated lecithin (breaks down bumps or cholesterol under the skin)
½–1 tbsp. honey
1–2 sliced bananas (any fresh fruit can be substituted)

Mix in blender. (Add 3–4 ice cubes for thicker shake.)

or

HONEY HEAVEN

(A warm quick drink, and my son Evan's favorite)

1 cup skim (or low-fat) milk
1 tsp. honey
¾ tsp. vanilla
cinnamon

Warm milk, honey, and vanilla, then pour quickly in blender to froth. Serve and sprinkle with cinnamon. (One serving supplies approximately 8 g. of protein and 300 mg. of calcium. A nice way to start any day.)

Do you consider whole wheat pancakes a nutritious breakfast?
They are nutritious in that three average pancakes contain approximately 7 g. of protein (the equivalent of 1 egg) and those made with buttermilk have even more protein. Whole wheat has more fiber than refined flour, and may help in the prevention of constipation, diverticulosis, and colon cancer. On the other hand,

pancakes, particularly in convenience mixes, are high in sodium. Three pancakes provide anywhere between 500 mg. and 1,000 mg. of sodium, which would negate their nutritional value for anyone concerned about their sodium intake.

Also, you have to realize that pancakes are usually adorned with butter and syrup, adding more sodium, fat, and sugar. But if you make your own pancakes, cook them on a non-stick griddle that requires no extra grease, add minimum salt, eat two instead of three, and go lightly on the syrup, they're a fine way to start the day.

Could you please tell me the differences between cereals labeled "fiber rich," "high fiber," and "more fiber"?

It depends on the cereal in most cases. Because the FDA hasn't ruled that cereals must have a certain amount of fiber in order to make their label claims, the hype is up (or down) for grabs.

As a rule, if a cereals claims to be a "good fiber source," it contains 2 g. per ounce serving; if the claim is "fiber rich" it has 4 g.; for "maximum fiber" it has 9 g. On the other hand, rules don't always apply. For example, "More Fiber" means 12 g. for General Mills' Fiber One, but only 5 g. for Post Natural Bran Flakes. And 5 g. means "High Fiber" if you're buying Ralston Bran Chex, but 9 g. if you purchase Kellogg's All Bran. If you really want to know the differences, ignore the bold print on the front of the boxes and read the small print on the sides.

Do breads that are made with alpha-cellulose really have more fiber than whole wheat breads?

Yes they do, but it's not the fiber you want (see section 101). Alpha-cellulose is nothing more than wood pulp. It can give a bread 400 percent more fiber than a whole wheat competitor, but there is no indication that it may help prevent colon cancer. If you want to increase your fiber intake, there are much better ways than eating sawdust.

4

COFFEE, TEA, OR MILK?

42. That Not-So-Great Cup of Coffee

A lot of bad things have been said about coffee, and with good reason.

Caffeine is one of the world's most psychoactive drugs.

The "lift" you get from coffee that brings about an almost immediate sense of clearer thought and increased energy comes from the release of sugar stored in the liver. This is caused by caffeine, a central nervous system stimulant also present in tea, colas, chocolate, and some medications (see section 47). But it's an upper with a lot of downers:

• As few as 3 or 4 cups of coffee daily can cause psychological and physical addiction.
• Depending on the amount consumed, or individual insensitivity, it can cause a condition known as caffeinism, with symptoms of appetite loss, irritability, insomnia, headaches, heart palpitations, irritation of the stomach, diarrhea, nausea, increased urination, anxiety attacks, flushing, chills, and sometimes a low fever.
• The release of stored sugar places heavy stress on the endocrine system.

• Caffeine's diuretic properties put extra stress on the kidneys and have a dehydrating effect on the body.

• Various studies have linked caffeine consumption to birth defects and the Center for Science in the Public Interest advises pregnant women to avoid it.

• The *American Journal of Obstetrics and Gynecology* reports that women who consume more than 150 mg. of caffeine a day during pregnancy are more likely than those who consume less (or none at all) to miscarry between the third and seventh months of gestation.

• Effects of caffeine wear off less quickly on pregnant women and women on the Pill, taking about twice as long to clear out from their systems.

• Coffee increases the acidity in your gastrointestinal tract and can cause rectal itching.

• Drinking coffee to wake up in the morning can reset your body's circadian clock, interfere with your natural A.M. adrenaline, and cause a phase-delay similar to jet lag that can result in unexplainable drowsiness, depression, and insomnia, later on or the next day.

• Excessive intake of methylxanthines, a group of compounds to which caffeine belongs (and which includes theophylline, found in tea, and theobromine, found in chocolate), has been linked to fibrocystic breast disease and prostate problems.

• The British medical journal *Lancet* has reported a strong relationship between coffee consumption and cancer of the bladder and the lower urinary tract.

• Caffeine has been found to interfere with DNA replication.

• Recent studies at Stanford University have found that drinking 2 to 3 cups of strong coffee a day is associated with elevated cholesterol levels.

• People who drink 5 cups of coffee daily have a 50 percent greater chance of having heart attacks than non–coffee drinkers.

• Two cups of coffee can raise blood pressure about an hour after consumption, as well as decrease, then increase, heart rate.

• Caffeine can rob the body of B vitamins, vitamin C, zinc, potassium, and other minerals, as well as prevent the proper absorption of iron; five (6-ounce) cups drunk within three hours can seriously deplete the body's supply of thiamine.

• Caffeine concentrations in breast milk often rise above those in the mother's blood, frequently causing crankiness, insomnia, colic, and other symptoms of caffeinism in nursing infants.

• More than moderate caffeine consumption, over 300 mg. daily, is inadvisable; excessive consumption, 1,000 mg. (approximately 10 cups of coffee) daily, is risky; toxicity varies with individuals, but 10 g. are estimated as the lethal dose.

• Abrupt abstention can cause mild to severe withdrawal symptoms.

43. The Dangers of Decaffeination

Just when you thought it was safe to drink coffee again, because each 5-ounce cup of brewed decaf contains only 3 mg. of caffeine instead of regular's 115 mg., you find your health jeopardized by something even more sinister: methylene chloride.

An acknowledged animal carcinogen (linked to liver and lung cancers), whose use the FDA has already proposed banning in hairsprays, methylene chloride remains the most widely used solvent for the extraction of caffeine from coffee beans. Though manufacturers claim that the solvent evaporates after the beans are steamed, heated, and blown dry, an uncertain amount of harmful residue is suspected of remaining. The FDA is currently investigating this, but methylene chloride is still being used to decaffeinate coffees that are being sold. And the labels don't say which ones!

44. Other Decaffeinators

There are safer, though more expensive, alternatives to decaffeinating coffee. But products using them are well worth the price. Ethyl acetate, a natural derivative of coffee and other fruits, such as bananas and pineapples, is used to extract caffeine. The process takes more time, but the results are the same, only safer. Most teas use ethyl acetate for decaffeination.

Your wisest choice is to select brands that have been decaffeinated by the Swiss water process. No chemicals are used in soaking the beans, which are later passed through activated charcoal or carbon filters to remove the caffeine. Products decaffeinated by the Swiss water process will usually say so; it's a sales plus that manufacturers can be proud of.

45. Withdrawal Warning

Weaning yourself from caffeine is not easy. In fact, studies have shown that heavy coffee drinkers can experience withdrawal symptoms 12 to 16 hours after their last dose of caffeine, even if they've drunk decaf during that time period. The cutback in caffeine is substantial (see section 47 for comparisons) and the symptoms unpleasant.

But unpleasant as they are, if they're unrecognized for *what* they are, they can be confused with symptoms of other ailments, often resulting in misdiagnoses and unnecessary treatments. This does not mean that you should assume they are due to caffeine withdrawal and therefore ignore them. But if they coincide with your cutting back on caffeine, or making any dietary changes, your doctor should be informed.

COMMON CAFFEINE WITHDRAWAL SYMPTOMS MOST PEOPLE ARE NOT AWARE OF

• Headaches (eliminating a habitual after-dinner cup can cause morning headache the next day; tension headaches are often caused by recurrent caffeine withdrawal; holiday and weekend headaches occur frequently in office workers used to regular coffee breaks during their workweek)
• Irritability (sudden anger, intolerance of ordinary occurrences, frustration)
• Depression (moodiness, bouts of crying, general apathy, disinterest in work and hobbies, social withdrawal)
• Runny nose
• Nausea, queasiness, and vomiting (intermittent, frequently confused with stomach viruses)
• Fatigue (yawning, drowsiness)
• Dizziness

Easing up on caffeine should be done gradually. (A good way to start is by brewing equal parts regular and decaf, then increasing the proportion of decaf to regular.) Though some people can do it in a day or two with no repercussions, most require at least two weeks.

46. Coffee Trade-offs

There are two main species of coffee beans—*Coffea arabica* and *Coffea robusa*. Arabicas have approximately half the caffeine content of robustas, and fortunately, are the beans most often sold in supermarkets and specialty stores. (Most decaffeinated coffees are made from robustas because they provide a larger amount of caffeine for resale to manufacturers of soft drinks and drugs.)

INSTEAD OF...	SWITCH TO...
Regular coffee	"Light coffee" (a blend of wheat or chicory and coffee, with a generally lower caffeine content)
Drip coffee	Percolated (has approximately 30 mg. less caffeine)
Percolated coffee	Instant (has approximately 15 mg. less caffeine)
Instant coffee	Brewed decaffeinated (has approximately 62 mg. less caffeine)
Brewed decaffeinated coffee	Instant decaffeinated (has approximately 63 mg. less caffeine)
Instant decaffeinated coffee	Grain beverages, such as Postum or Pero (which are sort of imitation coffees made from bran, wheat, and molasses), or Cafix (made from barley, rye, chicory, and beets), have no caffeine. (**CAUTION:** Though these grain products are low in calories and caffeine free, excessive consumption may have an unwanted laxative effect or cause flatulence.)

If you crave a caffeine lift but want to avoid caffeine consequences, try ginseng (see section 117) or fruit juice, whose natural sugar content can give you an energy boost—with a vitamin bonus.

47. Caffeine Comparisons to Keep in Mind

The following table has been designed to give perspective to caffeine consumption and help you keep yours at a safe 300 mg. daily. You're likely to find that you are getting more caffeine jolts than you think.

COFFEE	PER 5-OUNCE SERVING
Dripolated	110–150 mg.
Percolated	64–124 mg.
Instant	40–108 mg.
Light coffee-grain blend	12–35 mg.
Decaffeinated	2–5 mg.
Instant decaffeinated	2 mg.

TEA	PER 5-OUNCE SERVING
Black 5-minute brew	20–50 mg.
Green 5-minute brew	35 mg.
Black 3-minute brew	20–46 mg.
Black 1-minute brew	9–33 mg.
Instant	12–28 mg.
Iced	22–36 mg.
Decaffeinated (see section 48)	10–41 mg.

CHOCOLATE	
Cocoa (5-ounce cup)	4–6 mg.
Milk chocolate (1 ounce)	5–6 mg.
Dark chocolate, semisweet (1 ounce)	20–35 mg.

SOFT DRINKS	PER 12-OUNCE SERVING
Jolt Cola	74 mg.
Mountain Dew	54 mg.
Mello Yello	52 mg.
Diet Mr. Pibb	52 mg.
Tab	46 mg.
Coca-Cola	46 mg.
Diet Coke	46 mg.
Shasta Cola	46 mg.
Dr. Pepper	44 mg.
Pepsi-Cola	41 mg.
Diet Pepsi	38 mg.
RC Cola	36 mg.
Mr. Pibb	33 mg.
7UP	0 mg.
Root beer	0 mg.
Ginger ale	0 mg.
Decaffeinated colas	trace
Tonic water	0 mg.
Club soda, seltzer	0 mg.

DRUGS	PER TABLET
Vivarin	200 mg.
Bio Slim T Capsules	140 mg.
Aqua-Ban	100 mg.
Cafergot	100 mg.
NoDoz	100 mg.
Excedrin	65 mg.
(Excedrin P.M. has no caffeine but does have an antihistamine)	
Fiorinal	40 mg.
Vanquish	33 mg.
Anacin	32 mg.
Darvon Compound	32 mg.
Empirin	32 mg.
Midol	32 mg.
Soma Compound	32 mg.
Triaminicin	30 mg.
Aspirin	0 mg.

48. The Tea Alternatives

The amount of caffeine in tea varies according to the type of leaves and the strength of the brew. The longer tea steeps, the more caffeine it will have. The average cup has about half the caffeine of coffee, and loose teas contain much less than those made with tea bags.

Be forewarned that decaffeinated teas still contain some caffeine. Lipton decaffeinated tea has only 10 mg., but Salada has 41 mg. For caffeine-sensitive individuals, three or more cups daily could cause adverse reactions.

All herbal teas contain no caffeine, but the same is not true of all flavored teas, or herbal-flavored teas. Celestial Seasonings Morning Thunder, for instance, whose flavor is derived from mate (a South American plant whose leaves are rich in caffeine) and other tea leaves, contains 35 mg. of caffeine. Flavored black teas (orange, cinnamon, blackberry, apple, and so forth) contain about the same amount, which is still less than unflavored black teas. Some decaffeinted flavored teas, such as those made by Bromley and Benchley, have about 24 mg. per tea bag.

Herbal teas make fine, caffeine-free alternatives to coffee, but they do have other hazards that you should be aware of. (See section 104.)

49. What Could Be Wrong with Milk?

A lot if—

• You're an adult concerned about your fat consumption, because whole milk has 65 percent saturated fatty acids and only 4 percent polyunsaturates.

• You or a member of your family has a lactose intolerance (a deficiency of the enzyme lactase necessary for milk digestion), which can cause such gastrointestinal problems as bloating, cramps, and diarrhea; or a milk allergy (hypersensitivity to the protein in milk), which can cause reactions such as eczema, asthma, ear infections, excessive fatigue, diarrhea, or constipation, among others, and are frequently mistaken for symptoms of other health problems.

• You are concerned about arteriosclerosis (an acknowledged precursor to heart attacks), because the fatty particles in homogenized whole milk can pass through the stomach wall into the bloodstream, making arteries susceptible to cholesterol buildup.

• The FDA does not ban the use of BGH (Bovine Growth Hormone), which increases milk production but can leave potentially harmful residues in milk.

• You have stomach acidity problems or ulcers. New studies show that milk (whole, low-fat, and skim) stimulates gastric acid secretions and aggravates rather than soothes ulcerative or pre-ulcerative conditions.

• You have hypertension or cardiovascular disease and want to keep your sodium intake in check. Milk and all milk products, with the exception of low-sodium milk and cheeses, are high sodium suppliers.

• Your children drink it in place of other, iron-rich foods. Overconsumption of cow's milk, a poor source of iron, can cause microscopic losses of blood from the gastrointestinal tract and lead to iron deficiency anemia.

• The milk is raw (unpasteurized), because it may contain dangerous microorganisms that could cause serious illness, and be potentially lethal for infants and young children.

• It has an off-flavor that could be caused by cow feed sprayed with harmful pesticides.

• You rely on it as your sole source of calcium. Adults and growing children need 800 to 1,200 mg. of calcium daily. Three 8-ounce glasses of whole milk will give you only 776 mg. of calcium—not enough and certainly not worth the 360 mg. of sodium, 33 mg. of cholesterol, 15 g. of saturated fat, and 577 calories you'll get with them. Exchanging whole milk for skim or low-fat milk, or buttermilk, will cut back calories and fat, but still won't provide enough calcium. (See section 128 for additional sources.)

50. Milk Trade-offs

IF YOU HAVE A LACTOSE INTOLERANCE

• Acidophilus milk (uses safe bacterial cultures, such as those in cheeses, yogurt, and sour cream, to predigest the lactose).

• Buttermilk (made with skim or low-fat pasteurized milk to which a bacterial culture that predigests lactose is added).

• Sweet acidophilus milk (bacterial cultures are added, but don't break down the lactose until the milk enters your digestive tract). This milk cannot be warmed, used for cooking, or added to hot liquids.

• Lactase-treated milk, which can be made by adding 4 to 5 drops of the liquid enzyme lactase (available at health stores and pharmacies as LACT-AID) to a quart of milk. This sweetens the milk, but adds no calories or carbohydrates, and the treated milk can be used any way that you would use ordinary milk.

IF YOU HAVE A MILK ALLERGY

• Soy milks (available in health food stores).

• Any dairy products marked "parve"; these are milk free.

TO MINIMIZE CHOLESTEROL AND SATURATED FAT

• Skim milk (4 mg. cholesterol, .28 g. saturated fat per cup).

• Buttermilk (9 mg. cholesterol, 1.3 g. saturated fat per cup).

• Mix 2 percent milk with skim milk (you will get a lot more taste and only a little more cholesterol and fat).

• Use sour cream instead of heavy cream.

• Use sour half-and-half, or low-fat yogurt, instead of sour cream.

TO MINIMIZE SODIUM

• Low-sodium milk (95 percent of the sodium has been removed).

FOR THE CREAM IN YOUR COFFEE

• Mix equal parts whole and skim milk; better yet, equal parts low-fat (or 2 percent) and skim milk.

51. Never Trust a Non-dairy Creamer

Keep your glasses with you when you shop so that you can read the small print on non-dairy creamer labels. You'll be in for quite a few surprises.

• Though these "creamers" don't contain lactose, almost all contain sodium caseinate, a derivative of milk protein that can cause reactions in people with milk allergies. Moreover, the processing used to produce sodium caseinate results in the formation of some lysinoalanine (LAL), which is under investigation for being a factor in causing kidney damage, and, if spray-dried, may also result in the formation of nitrites (see section 35). Additionally, tests to determine whether caseinates can cause birth defects have not yet been conducted.

• Non-dairy does not mean either "low calorie" or "unsaturated fat." Despite their lack of butterfat, the primary fat source in these "creamers" is almost always a highly saturated vegetable oil (such as coconut oil, which is more saturated than most animal fats) that supplies as many calories and usually even more saturated fat than whole milk.

• Many non-dairy creamers also contain carrageenan (see section 24), an additive of dubious safety that you are wise to avoid.

• No non-dairy creamers have any nutritional value worth mentioning, and can contain up to 68 percent sugar.

• Liquid creamers usually have more calories per serving, but generally have substantially lower levels of saturated fat.

• A few non-dairy creamers use soy protein instead of sodium caseinate, but beware of those that merely claim to contain a nonspecific vegetable protein.

52. Any Questions About Chapter 4?

I drink low-fat milk all the time and have gotten to the point where it tastes the same as whole milk to me—except in my coffee. Does the coffee cause the milk to change?

No, it's the other way around. A milk's fat content produces the change in coffee's color (the reflection of light from homogenized fat globules causes the coffee to look lighter). It is essentially an optical effect. If someone else adds the milk to your coffee, and you don't look at it before you drink it, you'll find that you no longer taste the difference.

5

THE LUNCH CRUNCH

53. Dying for Lunch?

Two heart attacks occur every minute in the United States. The top nutritional culprits, according to a recent study conducted by the Department of Health and Human Services, are fat, cholesterol, sodium, and sugar.

> Your idea of a prudent diet might be killing you.

This probably comes as no great surprise to anyone who hasn't been secluded on a desert island for the last ten years, but the fact that what most people think of as a prudent diet is so far from one as to be deadly, should be enough to shock everyone. And I certainly hope that it does.

If you think you have cut your risk of cancer and heart disease just because you no longer eat butter or use cream, have virtually eliminated fried foods from your diet, trim the fat from your meat, drink diet sodas, and haven't had bacon or sausage with your eggs for years, you are fooling yourself and foiling your health. *It's not so much a matter of what you do or don't eat, but rather how often you do or don't eat it that matters!*

54. Packing Lunch Boxes with Trouble

White bread and rolls (see section 39) provide large portions of unwanted nutrients because we eat them so often. But they are the frame for sandwiches (very few people brown-bag salads for lunch) and account for 22.3 percent of a combined fat, sodium, and sugar intake before we even put anything on them.

Since bread alone does not a sandwich make, add *just 2 ounces* of any of the following and you'll have a pretty good idea of what else you're getting:

FILLING	FAT	SODIUM
Bologna	11 g.	737 mg.
Ham	17 g.	476 mg.
Turkey (light meat)	2.2 g.	42 mg.
Swiss cheese	15.6 g.	148 mg.
American Cheddar	18.8 g.	352 mg.
Peanut butter	36 g.	298 mg.
Tunafish (water)	less than 1 g.	216 mg.

Add a tablespoon of mayo, butter, or margarine and you'll have another 11 g. of fat. (That's also 140 mg. of sodium if you use butter or margarine; mayo has only 14 mg.) A tablespoon of mustard and ketchup, on the other hand, will spare you the fat, but the mustard will give you 195 mg. of sodium and the ketchup an equally substantial 156 mg., as well as more sugar than an equivalent portion of ice cream!

Also keep in mind that with the exception of bratwurst, virtually all luncheon meats, frankfurters, knockwurst, and other processed meats, as well as smoked fish, contain nitrates and nitrites (see section 35).

55. Sandwich Cautions

Stocking up on fillings, or preparing sandwiches beforehand so you can get the kids off to school or yourself off to work in time, is a fine idea, providing you keep a few things in mind.

SANDWICH SAFETY

• Even if refrigerated, don't keep uncured luncheon meats for more than 4 to 7 days. (If they get that shiny, slimy look, toss them out.)

• When making sandwiches with uncured meats, don't let them stand unrefrigerated for more than 5 to 10 minutes. (Rewrap and refrigerate quickly to prevent bacterial growth.)

• If you are making chicken, egg, or tunafish salad, refrigerate immediately after adding the mayonnaise. (The mayo itself doesn't spoil, but when combined with tuna, chicken, hard boiled eggs, or meat, it can become a bacterial spawning ground.) You can keep the sandwich cold until lunchtime by packing it with a box of frozen juice or a "blue ice" pack.

• If making a sliced egg or egg salad sandwich, be sure you don't cook and then let the unshelled eggs cool in water. (Cooling eggs in water causes them to lose their natural protective layer and sets up a breeding ground for a bacteria that produces a nerve-damaging toxin. And if they are *then* stored in airtight containers, even more toxins are produced.) The best way to cool boiled eggs is to let them stand in the open air and then refrigerate.

• Make sandwiches on frozen bread. This will keep the filling cool and the sandwich tasting freshly made when lunchtime arrives.

• Sandwiches can be made beforehand and frozen (wrapped in foil) until needed. But lettuce and other greens should not be frozen. They can be added when the sandwich is taken out of the freezer.

56. The Scoop on School Lunches
School lunches, though nutritionally balanced *in theory*, are *in fact* so nutritionally poor (with very few exceptions) that they are virtually hazardous to a growing child's health.

Schools can teach children some of the worst nutritional habits.

Though lunches served in school are required to provide at least one-third of a child's daily recommended nutrient allowance (by including milk, a protein-rich food, fruit, vegetables, a grain food, and butter or margarine), they rarely do. Most of the meals are low in fiber, high in refined carbohydrates and sugars, and surfeited with processed, vitamin-depleted foods. And adding insult to nutritional injury, the food tastes awful, too, as evidenced by what gets tossed in the lunchroom garbage.

Additionally, many schools have vending machines for gum, soft drinks, and other junk foods, which compound the problem by teaching children poor nutritional habits right in their halls of learning.

The convenience of having a child eat lunch at school is not worth the nutritional cost. A high-sugar intake at lunch can cause a drop in blood sugar during the afternoon, which can in turn leave a child fatigued, inattentive, and unable to retain what is being taught. Refined sugar has also been linked to delinquency. (See section 134.)

57. Simple Sandwiches for Superior Performance

It is easier than you think to prepare nutritious lunches for your child and yourself without having to resort to expensive, non-nutritive processed luncheon meats.

SEVEN SUPER SANDWICH LUNCHES YOU CAN PACK IN PLAIN BROWN BAGS

1. Cottage cheese and pineapple (unsweetened) sandwich on nut-bread/carrot sticks/sunflower seeds/low-fat milk.

2. Tuna salad with lettuce in pita bread/cherry tomatoes/pear or peach/low-fat milk. (*Hint:* Yogurt can be used instead of mayo for making tuna just as good, and it has much less fat.)

3. Ricotta (or cottage) cheese and raisin sandwich on banana bread/green pepper slices/tangerine/low-fat milk.

4. Peanut butter and sliced apple sandwich/carrot sticks/orange slices/low-fat milk.

5. Chicken salad with chopped celery in pita bread/apple/low-fat milk.

6. Baked beans (mashed with a little onion and homemade chili sauce) in pita bread/cucumber strips/melon slices or cubes/low-fat milk.

7. Chopped egg (mixed with a little mayo or yogurt, grated onion and carrot) on oat bread/peanuts/grapes/low-fat milk.

58. Fast-food Foolishness

Lunch is the meal most people eat away from home, and eating at fast-food restaurants has become a national pastime, as well as a shortcut to widespread health problems.

> If you think the four major food groups are McDonald's, Burger King, Pizza Hut, and Wendy's, you are in trouble.

I'm not condemning fast foods as nutritional wipeouts. They have a few (and I mean a *few*) redeeming features, primarily protein (see section 91). And an occasional burger and fries (and I do mean *occasional*) is unlikely to cause any serious repercussions for most people. But if you think that the four major food groups are McDonald's, Burger King, Pizza Hut, and Wendy's, you are in trouble.

The biggest problem with fast foods is their abundance of saturated fat and sodium. Since heart disease is the nation's number-one killer, the fact that most fast-food chains still fry their food in shortening that is largely beef tallow (it's hard to get fat more saturated than that) and have excessive amounts of salt in everything, is undeniably scary.

Consumers are generally unaware of how much fat and sodium they are getting because they don't expect it in things like shakes (Burger King's Vanilla has 9 g. of fat and 329 mg. of sodium) or apple pie (a slice of McDonald's has 19 g. of fat and 414 mg. of sodium). But it's there. And if you have a Whopper and fries with your Burger King shake you are getting a total of 51 g. of fat and 1,243 mg. of sodium—and that's without dipping your fries in ketchup (156 mg. of sodium per tablespoon) or sprinkling them with salt. No matter what your age or sex, that's more fat and sodium than your body can handle for lunch—or any single meal—on a regular basis.

59. Fast-food Calorie Countdown

BURGERS	CALORIES
Burger King Whopper	663
McDonald's Big Mac	587
Hardee's Big Deluxe	557
Wendy's Single (w/cheese)	547
Jack-in-the-Box Jumbo Jack (w/out cheese)	544
Arby's cheeseburger	492
Roy Rogers ¼ lb. (w/cheese)	416
Burger Chef Hamburger	258

CHICKEN	CALORIES
Kentucky Fried Chicken Extra Crispy Dinner (3 pieces of chicken)	950
(Original Recipe Dinner)	830
Jack-in-the-Box Chicken Supreme	572
Roy Rogers Fillet Sandwich	526
Wendy's Fillet Sandwich	441
Kentucky Fried Chicken Fillet Sandwich	399
McDonald's McNuggets (3¾ oz.)	286

FISH	CALORIES
Long John Silver's Fish Sandwich	560
Hardee's Big Fish	515
Burger King Whaler	502
Arthur Treacher's Fish Sandwich	440
McDonald's Fillet-O-Fish	373
Long John Silver's Fish (2 pieces)	318

Pizza and Tacos   Calories

Jack-in-the-Box Super Taco	375
Taco Bell Taco Light	372
Pizza Hut Thick 'N Chewy Pepperoni Pizza (¼ of 10 in. pie)	280
Pizza Hut Thin 'N Crispy Cheese Pizza (¼ of 10 in. pie)	225
Taco Bell Taco	194
Jack-in-the-Box Taco	174

Other Entrees   Calories

Arby's Roast Beef Sandwich	416
Roy Rogers Ham/Swiss	416
McDonald's Egg McMuffin	352
Dairy Queen Cheese Dog	330
Hardee's Chili Dog	329
Wendy's Chili (small)	310
Roy Rogers Roast Beef Sandwich	298

Fries (small)   Calories

Wendy's	317
Long John Silver's	282
McDonald's	268
Roy Rogers	230
Kentucky Fried Chicken	221
Jack-in-the-Box	217
Hardee's	202
Arby's	195
Burger King	158

Chocolate Shakes   Calories

Roy Rogers	518
McDonald's	377
Burger King	367
Wendy's	367

CHOCOLATE SHAKES	CALORIES
Arby's	365
Jack-in-the-Box	324
Hardee's	273

60. Some Fast-food Fat Trade-offs

If you're going to eat fast foods, you might want to give some heartfelt thought to choosing the lesser of their fatty evils.

INSTEAD OF . . .	CONSIDER PERHAPS . . .
Kentucky Fried Chicken Extra Crispy Dinner (3 pieces of chicken), which contains 54 g. fat	Pizza Hut Thin 'N Crispy Cheese Pizza (¼ of 10 in. pie), which contains 7.5 g. fat
A Burger King Whaler with 46 g. fat	Two pieces of Long John Silver's Fish with 19 g. fat
A McDonald's Big Mac with 31 g. fat	A Burger Chef Hamburger with 13 g. fat, or a Taco Bell Taco with only 8 g. fat
Cheeseburgers	Regular burgers
Fries	Coleslaw
Fried clams, shrimp, or oysters	Large pieces of fish (which have more food in proportion to batter); or even better, broiled fish
Fried chicken	Broiled chicken; or removing the batter-fried skin
Shakes	Fruit juice

In all cases, you should learn to balance fast-food indulgences with a subsequent meal containing fresh fruit, green and yellow vegetables, whole grains, beans, and foods that are rich in vitamins A, C, the B complex, and iron. (For a list of best sources, see section 128.)

61. Not So Hot Dogs
Hot dogs might have made Nathan's famous, but they won't do much for you.

A HOT DOG BY ANY NAME IS STILL NOT SO HOT

• Its main ingredient is the scraps and trimmings of muscle meat, usually beef and pork (unless otherwise stated), but not necessarily in equal proportions or in that order.
• It is high in saturated fats.
• It consists primarily of water and fat: approximately 56 percent water and 26 percent fat.
• Its protein content is approximately 13 percent.
(To give you an idea of how little protein you are getting for your fat and your dollar, cooked steak and hamburger have approximately 25 percent protein. The protein in ground sirloin costs about $12.50 a pound; the protein in the average hot dog costs about $14.50 per pound.)
• It may contain 3½ percent of nonmeat-nonwater ingredients, usually substances such as calcium-reduced dried skim milk, which are used as binders.
• It contains preservatives and flavorings, such as salt, sweeteners, ascorbic acid, sodium erythorbate or ascorbate, and nitrite. As explained in section 35, nitrites can form nitrosamines, which have been found to be carcinogenic. (There is no such thing as a nitrite-free hot dog, since those look-alikes that are nitrite free must be labeled "uncured cooked sausage.")
• Sodium content ranges from 300 mg. (Best's Kosher Beef Lower Fat hot dog) to 645 mg. (Hygrade's Beef hot dog).

MY ADVICE: The next time you decide you want to eat a hot dog, change your mind.

62. Any Questions About Chapter 5?

What's the worst thing about fast foods?

Aside from people eating them too often, they contain too much protein, salt, fat, and calories and not enough complex carbohydrates and fiber. One typical fast-food meal (cheeseburger, fries, and shake) can supply 90 percent of your daily protein, and often a day's worth of fat, salt, and calories as well. This leaves little leeway for healthful eating, and plenty of room for extra pounds of trouble.

My husband is a truck driver, and he eats a lot of fast foods, even though he sometimes develops a rash after eating them. Do you know what causes this? And are there any vitamins that can help?

A lot of fast-food ingredients can trigger allergic reactions in sensitive individuals. Along with such additives as Yellow Food Dye No. 5 (often in hotcakes and milk shakes), corn sugar (frequently in french fries), and milk solids (used in fish fillet), MSG is probably the most frequent culprit. It has been known to cause rashes, itches, and insomnia in individuals with no previous allergies or food sensitivities. And most fast-food restaurants use MSG, particularly in soups, but also in burgers and other foods.

Another possibility could be sulfites, which though now banned from being sprayed on fresh vegetables, are still used in frozen ones, soups, potato salad, gravies, beer, and foods commonly served at diners and fast-food restaurants. (See section 28.)

I'd suggest your husband take a high-potency multiple vitamin and mineral twice daily (with meals), along with vitamin C, 500 mg., vitamin E, 200–400 mg., and vitamin B complex 50–100 mg. I would also advise lecithin, either 3 tablespoons of granules or 12 capsules daily. And considering his eating habits, one multiple digestive enzyme daily is also recommended.

6
SCARY SNACKS

63. The Unsweet Side of Sugar

We are eating 11 more pounds of sugar, or its equivalent, than we did ten years ago, when we were eating 118.1 pounds of it annually! What's worse is that most of us don't even know it.

All carbohydrate sweeteners qualify as sugar, even though they may be called by other names (see section 10). Sugar not only sweetens, it also acts as a preservative, and retains and absorbs moisture. It is often found in products we wouldn't think contained it: salt, peanut butter, canned vegetables, bouillon cubes, medicines, toothpaste, vitamins, and more.

WHAT IT CAN DO TO YOU

- Cause tooth decay.
- Contribute to obesity.
- Aggravate asthma, mental illness, and nervous disorders.
- Cause personality changes and mood swings.
- Increase the possibility of heart disease, diabetes, hypertension, gallstones, back problems, arthritis, hypoglycemia, and other ailments.
- Cause loss of essential nutrients.
- Potentiate salt to raise blood pressure.
- Imbalance the body's calcium/phosphorous ratio.

64. A Table of Sugar Contents

With sugar, it is definitely a matter of hide-and-sweet, since manufacturers know that its presence is not desired by consumers. Yet
sugar, which provides none of the forty-four nutrients needed to
sustain life, accounts for more than 24 percent of the calories the
average American consumes daily, whether he or she knows it or
not.

FOOD	SERVING SIZE	APPROXIMATE TEASPOONS OF SUGAR PER SERVING
DRINKS		
Birds Eye Awake	4 oz.	3
Canada Dry Tonic Water	12 oz.	18¼
Chocolate milk	8 oz.	6
Cola beverages	6 oz.	3½
Eggnog	8 oz.	8
Ginger ale	6 oz.	5
Grapefruit juice (unsweetened)	4 oz.	2½
Hi-C Orange Drink	6 oz.	5
Kool-Aid	8 oz.	6
Malted milk shake	10 oz.	5
Orangeade	8 oz.	5
Orange juice	4 oz.	2½
Root beer	10 oz.	4½
7-Up	6 oz.	3¾
Tang	4 oz.	4
CANDIES		
Chewing gum	1 stick	½
Chocolate bar	1½ oz.	2½
Chocolate mints	1	2
Granola Clusters	1 oz.	3⅓
Gumdrop	1	2

Food	Serving Size	Approximate Teaspoons of Sugar Per Serving
CANDIES		
Hard candy	4 oz.	10
Lifesavers	1	1/3
Marshmallow	1 regular	1½
Milky Way	1 oz.	4
Peanut brittle	1 oz.	3½
CAKES, COOKIES, AND PIES		
Angel food	1 (4-oz. piece)	7
Apple pie	1 slice	12
Brownie	1 (¾ oz.)	3
Cheesecake	1 (4-oz. piece)	2
Cherry pie	1 slice	14
Chocolate cake (plain)	1 (4-oz. piece)	6
Chocolate cake (iced)	1 (4-oz. piece)	10
Chocolate cookie	1	1½
Chocolate éclair	1	7
Cream puff (iced)	1 regular	5
Cupcake (iced)	1	6
Doughnut (plain)	1	3
Doughnut (glazed)	1	6
Fig Newtons	1	5
Gingersnaps	1	3
Macaroons	1	6
Oatmeal cookies	1	2
Pumpkin pie	1 slice	10
Sponge cake	1 (4-oz. piece)	6
Sugar cookies	1	1½
FRUIT AND DAIRY DESSERTS		
Applesauce (unsweetened)	½ cup	2
Canned fruit cocktail	½ cup	5
Canned peaches in syrup	2 halves (1 tbsp. syrup)	3½

Food	Serving Size	Approximate Teaspoons of Sugar Per Serving
FRUIT AND DAIRY DESSERTS		
Chocolate pudding	½ cup	4
Ice cream cone	1	3½
Ice cream soda	1	5
Ice cream sundae	1	7
Sherbert	½ cup	9
Tapioca pudding	½ cup	3

65. Why Quick Pickups Let You Down

Simple sugars, which most candies are, require little metabolizing and enter your bloodstream quickly, giving you that much touted *lift*. But the catch is that your pancreas, the organ in charge of releasing insulin to process carbohydrates (starches and sugars) to keep blood sugar at a steady and healthy level, is caught off guard by the sudden surge of sugar, and, thinking it has more work to do than it has, releases too much insulin.

> That instant pickup from a candy bar is really a downer in disguise.

The result is an in-body processing error that lets you down the hard way: a drop in blood sugar, usually within the hour, that leaves you feeling less energetic, less alert, and more hungry and irritable than you were before.

66. All Sugars Aren't the Same

There is no doubt that a sugar by any name is still a sugar (even when it is called a carbohydrate), but that doesn't mean they are all the same, or hazard-free.

SUGAR REVIEWS THAT AIN'T SO SWEET

Sucrose

Refined white table sugar, granulated or powdered, made from either sugarcane or sugar beets. Though a disaccharide, meaning a double sugar (composed of glucose and fructose, in this case), it is totally lacking in protein, vitamins, and minerals. The B vitamins needed for its assimilation must be obtained from other foods or supplements; when ample B vitamins are not supplied, they are taken from the body and can cause deficiencies.

Glucose

The body's blood sugar, glucose is also found in most fruits. It's a monosaccharide, the simplest form of sugar in which a carbohydrate is assimilated. It is rapidly assimilated and can upset blood sugar balance in the same way as sucrose, though it is only half as sweet. It is one of the basic sugars in sweeteners.

Dextrose

A monosaccharide that is chemically identical to glucose (which is frequently referred to as dextrose) and made from cornstarch.

Fructose

Also known as levulose, this is a natural sugar found in fruit. It is preferred to sucrose because it is absorbed more slowly into the body. But many fruits are mainly sucrose, so fructose should *not* be considered safe for diabetics or hypoglycemics. Additionally, the fructose used in foods is usually the result of enzymes added to corn syrup starch, which produces sucrose that is then further processed into a high fructose corn syrup. Even when derived solely from a natural source (which is rare because it is expensive), fructose is nonetheless a highly refined product and, like sugar, is devoid of nutrients.

Because fructose is sweeter than sucrose, and less is needed to obtain the same sweetness, it is often used in "lite" products to reduce calorie content by the necessary one-third. This has its advantages for weight watchers, but is not without drawbacks: Large amounts of fructose can cause diarrhea and gastrointestinal pain. It has also been found to cause a marked elevation in cholesterol levels.

Maltose

A disaccharide made from the malting of whole grains. (Sounds nutritious, but it isn't.) Though not nearly as sweet as either sucrose or fructose, maltose is much less likely to cause cavities.

Lactose

This is milk sugar, a combination of glucose and galactose, and the least sweet of all. Despite its derivation from milk, it is as non-nutritive as all other refined sugars, and can cause adverse reactions in individuals with a milk allergy or lactose intolerance. (See section 49.)

Brown Sugar

Plain old white, refined sugar with molasses coloring.

Raw Sugar
(Also known as "natural," blond, and turbinado)

All are simply white sugar, packaged at 96 percent sucrose; table sugar is bleached and purified to 99 percent. You might pay more for them, but you are still getting nothing but empty calories—and no nutritional benefits to offset the cost.

Blackstrap Molasses

The liquid that remains after beet or cane sugar has been thoroughly processed and the sucrose has been removed. Though still 65 percent sucrose, blackstrap molasses contains minor but useful amounts of iron, calcium, potassium, and B vitamins, particularly vitamin B_6. Lighter molasses is less endowed with nutrients.

CAUTION: If you are under levodopa treatment for Parkinson's disease, blackstrap molasses is not recommended.

Sorghum Molasses

One of the lighter molasseses, made from sweet sorghum (a cereal grass in the millet family). The juice is extracted from sorghum stalks through crushing and is then boiled down into syrup. It can be bought in this form, but unless the syrup is heated properly it may ferment in the jar quicky. Most manufacturers add enzymes to make it more stable and increase its shelf life. In any event, iron is the only significant nutrient, and the product is still about 65 percent sucrose.

Barbados Molasses

Another light molasses, processed the same way as sorghum, only sugarcane is used instead of sorghum. Its taste is much like blackstrap molasses, only more palatable, but it has virtually none of blackstrap molasses's nutrients. (NOTE: No molasses or any other sweetener made from sorghum or sugarcane is organic, since neither is a food crop and is frequently sprayed.)

Honey

This nectar of the gods is still sugar and has the highest sugar content of all natural sweeteners, approximately 65 calories per tablespoon. (Refined sugar has only 48 calories per tablespoon.) Honey does have small amounts of potassium, calcium, and phosphorus, which is more than you can say about refined sugar; and truly natural honey that is only heated to low temperatures (just enough to remove beeswax and other impurities) contains natural enzymes and pollen, a rich source of protein.

But consumers are being stung with honey rip-offs. Now that it has become popular with the health-conscious, manufacturers heat it to high temperatures to give it a crystal-clear purity that sells, but destroys nutrients. Some suppliers feed their bees sugar water, or worse, add sugar syrup to their honey for a better flavor.

The taste and color of honey should depend on the type of blossom from which it was gathered. Greek honey, for instance, comes from bees fed on thyme and has a distinct, though somewhat mediciney flavor. Irish honey, which comes from bees fed on heather, is mild. Buckwheat honey is dark, and unless you are really into honey, it is best used in bread-making. For flavoring beverages, clover or alfalfa honey is my choice. Blended honey is usually least distinctive, least expensive, and most likely to have no redeeming features.

Unfortunately, everything about honey isn't sweet. Aside from the fact that it can rot teeth faster than sucrose, various honeys have been found to contain carcinogens that the bees have extracted from flowers sprayed with cancer-causing pesticides. And some honeys (as well as corn syrups) can be fatal to infants whose digestive tracts aren't mature enough to prevent the growth of the botulinum spores that are occasionally present in these sweeteners.

Maple Syrup

If you want a naturally really sweet sweetener, pure maple syrup is one of the best, but it is expensive. Nonetheless, like molasses, maple syrup is still 65 percent sucrose, so no matter how much or little you pour on pancakes or French toast, approximately half is the equivalent of white sugar. Unfortunately, not all 100 percent pure maple syrup is 100 percent safe. Some producers don't make their maple syrup the old-fashioned way—by gathering the sap in lead-free buckets, boiling it down over hardwood fires, and bottling it. Instead, formaldehyde pellets are used to keep the tap holes from healing and increase sap flow. (Ingestion of formaldehyde, which is used in embalming fluids, can cause severe abdominal pain, internal bleeding, nausea, inability to urinate, coma, and death.) They also gather the sap in lead-soldered buckets. (The adverse effects of lead on infants and young children can occur at very low levels, causing symptoms ranging from mild anemia to severe brain damage and death.) Additionally, they boil the sap over oil fires, filter it, and add chemical antifoaming or polishing agents. Since all syrup tends to foam during processing, cream or animal fat has been used to reduce this, but some producers now use natural vegetable oil. (If you are a vegetarian or follow Jewish dietary laws and want to be sure the product contains no animal fat, check the ingredients or look for the word "parve" on the label.)

Malt Syrups

Nutritionally superior but not as sweet as maple syrups, the malt syrups are made from cereal grains (barley, rice, and wheat) and contain mainly maltose and glucose sugars. Keep in mind, though, that just because these syrups aren't as sweet as others doesn't mean they have a lower sugar content. Watch out for malt syrups that add sweetness with commercial corn syrup, which is industrially refined glucose.

The least sweet, but most wholesome, is 100 percent barley malt syrup. Rice syrup or rice honey, which is a mixture of barley and rice, comes in two types: one 20 percent barley and 80 percent rice, the other mostly rice with grain enzymes. Rice syrups are lighter in color and flavor but more costly. Quality malt syrups are made from simple sugars that have the least effect upon the body. Unfortunately, neither barley nor rice syrups are made from totally organic grains.

Xylitol

Though found naturally in berries, fruits, and mushrooms, it is produced commercially from "wood sugar," or xylose. Generally extracted from birch cellulose (a birchwood by-product of the plywood industry), it is considered a carbohydrate alcohol. It has the same caloric value as sugar, but is metabolized differently and therefore used in products for diabetics and hypoglycemics. Also, because bacteria in saliva don't grow on and ferment xylitol—as they do other sugars—to produce cavity-causing acids, it is used in many "sugar-free" chewing gums.

Until recently, the only known adverse effect of large doses has been diarrhea. But new studies show that large doses, in long-term feeding studies, have caused tumors and organ injury in animals; and humans receiving xylitol intravenously as an energy source have experienced liver, kidney, and brain disturbances. At this time it is under review by the FDA, and most U.S. manufacturers have voluntarily stopped using it. But not all "sugar-free" products are manufactured in the United States, so be sure to check labels.

Sorbitol

Half as sweet as sucrose, sorbitol (known as a sweet alcohol) occurs naturally in fruits, berries, algae, and seaweeds. But this is not from where manufacturers get it. It is made industrially from hydrogen and commercial glucose (corn sugar). Because of its slow absorption into the bloodstream, it is used in sugar-free gums (see section 68), candies, and other products okayed for use by diabetics and hypoglycemics. It does, though, have a laxative effect, and large doses (or frequent ingestion) generally cause diarrhea.

Mannitol

Much like sorbitol, this sweet alcohol occurs naturally in beets, celery, and olives, but is made industrially from hydrogen and glucose (corn sugar). Only half as sweet as sucrose, it is often used in powdered products, such as the dusting on chewing gum and breakfast cereals. It has a laxative effect at lower levels than sorbitol, and could produce diarrhea quite easily in infants and young children. Though it has been used as an additive in foods for over thirty years, there are no recorded long-term studies of its possible carcinogenic or mutagenic properties.

67. Real Facts About Artificial Sweeteners

Once upon a time, artificial sweeteners were used primarily by diabetics, who cannot adequately metabolize carbohydrates and for whom sugar can be lethal. Today, more than 70 million Americans, less than half of them diabetics, consume products containing sugar substitutes—none of which have been shown to be (at best) more than a partial aid to weight control and all of which pose health risks.

SACCHARIN

• One of the earliest, commercially used artificial sweeteners in the United States.
• A noncaloric petroleum derivative estimated to be 300 to 500 times sweeter than sugar, though it has a bitter aftertaste (which is now usually masked by the addition of the amino acid glycine).

• It is absorbed but not modified by the body, and is excreted unchanged in the urine.

• Studies have linked its use to bladder cancer in laboratory animals.

• The FDA proposed a ban on usage in 1977, but protests from consumers and the American Medical Association, the American Society of Internal Medicine, the National Academy of Sciences, the American Diabetes Association, and others called for a moratorium on the ban. The moratorium is still in effect while studies continue.

• As yet, no firm evidence has shown that saccharin causes cancer in humans, but warning labels informing consumers of the laboratory tests and the possibility of cancer must appear on products containing saccharin.

• Used in diet soft drinks, toothpaste, medicines, and available as the sugar substitute Sweet 'N Low.

• For diabetics, who must restrict carbohydrate intake, the risks of saccharin might be worth taking. For the general public, they are not.

CYCLAMATE

• Noncaloric and thirty times sweeter than sugar.

• Less expensive than either saccharin or aspartame, it is more effective when combined with either.

• It has been implicated in causing testicular atrophy and chromosome damage.

• Studies showing that when mixed with saccharin it increased the risk of bladder cancer caused it to be banned in the United States and Great Britain. (It is still used today in other countries.)

• Manufacturers are now petitioning the FDA to rescind the ban, on the basis that earlier tests were inconclusive, as opposed to presenting current proof of safety.

ASPARTAME

• Not technically an "artificial" sweetener because it is composed of two amino acids (phenylalanine and aspartic acid) that are natural components of many common proteins.

• Contains as many calories per gram as sugar (4 g.) but is about two hundred times sweeter, so much smaller amounts are needed.

• Considered safe by the FDA and the AMA except for persons suffering from PKU, an inherited inability to metabolize phenylalanine that can lead to severe retardation.

• Marketed as NutraSweet, it has replaced saccharin in almost all national soft drinks, with the exception of Dr. Pepper.

• It is used in an enormous variety of dietetic and low-calorie products, as well as medicines, and is available as the sugar substitute Equal.

• It has been implicated in numerous disorders, ranging from nausea and headaches to seizures, rashes, blindness, and brain damage.

• Phenylalanine can interfere with the body's chemical neurotransmitters that conduct nerve impulses within the brain. Therefore children who drink large quantities of diet sodas containing aspartame are particularly vulnerable to its dangerous side effects.

• Aspartame contains methyl or wood alcohol, which can affect fetal brain development. I would advise pregnant women who are watching their weight to avoid indulgence in diet products containing aspartame or any artificial sweetener.

68. What Four Out of Five Dentists Don't Tell You About Sugarless Gum

Four out of five dentists might recommend sugarless gum for their patients who chew gum, probably because they don't know what the fifth dentist does: that sugarless gum, or candy, can increase your chances of tooth decay if it contains sorbitol or mannitol—which most of them do.

Although neither sorbitol nor mannitol itself promotes cavities, both of them nourish and increase the type of bacteria in your mouth—namely, *Streptococcus mutans*—that do. According to Dr. Paul Keyes, founder of the International Dental Health Foundation, *Streptococcus mutans* have the mechanism to stick to teeth but will remain harmless until you eat something containing sugar or sucrose, with which they then quickly combine to cause decay. Because the sorbitol and mannitol have swelled the ranks of these bacteria, there are more of them available to use passing sugars to attack your teeth.

If you can't brush after every sweet, you can fight back by rinsing your mouth with water immediately (within 15 minutes) after eating or drinking anything that contains sucrose.

OTHER TOOTH-SAVING TIPS

• Eating aged cheese—cheddar or Swiss—can reduce the ability of plaque to form cavity-causing acids.

• Have your sweets *with* instead of *between* meals. (Sweets eaten with meals have little tendency to cause decay.)

• Be sure you are getting enough iron in your diet (see section 128), since sugars cause more damage to teeth if the body is deficient in iron.

• Increase your intake of fibrous foods (vegetables, whole-grain breads and pasta, cereals) which promote a stronger saliva flow and, essentially, "rinse" your teeth more frequently.

• Avoid excessive consumption of acidy fruit juices, which can wear away tooth enamel.

• Choose puddings or ice cream (which can be easily rinsed from the mouth) over caramels or fudge-type candies that stick to the teeth and are difficult to remove.

• If you are going to have a sweet, treat yourself and your teeth to a *small* piece of chocolate. Despite its multiple nutritive negatives, chocolate has been found to have decay-inhibiting properties.

• And try kissing more often. It stimulates the salivary glands, the saliva helps rinse food particles away, and, though it's not as effective as brushing or flossing, it's certainly more fun.

69. The Sweet Treat That Ought to Be Behind Bars

It is not difficult to become a chocoholic, but it is not healthy, either. In fact, chocolate's few benefits are far outweighed (in more ways than one) by its nutritional hazards.

THE GOOD CHIPS ABOUT CHOCOLATE

• It can help inhibit tooth decay. (Chocolate liquor, in chocolate candy, when mixed with sucrose, has been found to neutralize the effect of sucrose on the mouth's decay-causing bacteria, reducing their ability to produce cavity-causing acids.)

• It contains phenylethylamine, a natural mood-elavating substance that the brain produces when you are in love—and craves when you fall out of it.

NOW THE BAD . . .

• Chocolate, made from the cacao bean, contains significant amounts of caffeine (see section 42), which is an addictive drug.

• It is capable of depleting inositol, which aids in the redistribution of body fat, promotes healthy hair, and can help prevent eczema and keep cholesterol levels low.

• It can prevent the proper absorption of calcium, needed for the body's metabolization of iron, and therefore diminish energy, reflexes, bone strength and disease resistance, aggravate insomnia, and promote heartbeat irregularity.

• It can deplete the body of vitamin B_1 (thiamine) and other B vitamins needed for fighting stress and aiding in the digestion of carbohydrates.

• Its caffeine content can put heavy stress on the endocrine system, particularly a child's, and deplete necessary stores of potassium and zinc.

• It can delay the healing of canker sores.

• It is contraindicated for—and should definitely be avoided by—anyone who has herpes.

• It can worsen allergy symptoms and decrease the effectiveness of antihistamine medicines.

• It can decrease the effectiveness of tranquilizers, sedatives, and relaxants.

• It can cause serious hypertension in anyone taking a MAO inhibitor or an antidepressant.

• It has a large number of empty calories in small portions, making it easy to fill an empty stomach with too much fat and too few nutrients.

70. The Candy-*Candida* Connection

Yeast infections (*Candida albicans*) occur when the *Candida*, or yeast germ, gets out of control in the body, producing a toxin that not only affects the nervous system (causing headaches, fatigue, depression, hyperactivity, and memory loss, among other symptoms), but also the reproductive organs, leading to abdominal pain, persistent vaginitis, bladder problems, loss of sexual interest, and more.

Antibiotics, nutritional deficiencies, diabetes mellitus, birth control pills, cortisone, anxiety or physical stress, improper hygiene, chronic constipation or diarrhea, and food or chemical allergies are all possible causes of yeast infections, which are curable—provided you don't undermine the cure with the wrong foods.

Candida need certain foods to survive. This often causes patients suffering from yeast infections to have overwhelming cravings for sweets, which *Candida* thrive on. Giving in to these cravings will keep the *Candida* multiplying, along with producing uncomfortable side effects.

FOODS TO AVOID

Sugar, refined carbohydrates, all yeast-containing foods and any that may have mold. Particularly:

• Candy, ice cream, chocolate, chewing gum, colas, dried fruits
• Cheese, raised breads, sour cream, buttermilk
• Beer, wine, cider, soy sauce, vinegar, frozen or canned juices
• Mushrooms, tofu, melons

FOODS TO INCREASE

Some foods are natural combatants for yeast infections, and increasing them in your diet can help. Among them are garlic, onions, broccoli, cabbage, plain yogurt, turnips and other vegetables.

A HELPFUL SUPPLEMENT REGIMEN

- High-potency multiple vitamin, A.M. and P.M.
- High-potency chelated multiple minerals (with at least 1,000 mg. calcium and 500 mg. magnesium, as well as adequate amounts of iron, zinc, and selenium)
    - Vitamin C, 1,000 mg. (time release), A.M. and P.M.
    - Vitamin E (dry form), 200–400 IU, daily
    - Propolis, 500 mg., 3 times daily
    - Free-form amino acids (balanced formula) daily. (Take for at least several weeks or until the infection is gone.)

71. Little Snacks Can Have Big Dangers

There is no harm in having a snack or two now and then, unless you think of *now* as today and *then* as tomorrow, and wind up having one or more daily.

Even the calories in little snacks add up quickly. Just one pack of Lifesavers, eaten every day, can put 10 pounds on you in a year. And there's a lot more to being overweight than not fitting into your old jeans.

OBESITY

- Shortens life expectancy.
- Increases the risk of diabetes, heart attacks, strokes, gout, respiratory diseases, arthritis, and more.
- Has been found to be a factor in female infertility, menstrual disorders, toxemia, and various forms of cancer.
- Can delay wound healing, lower resistance to infection, and generally undermine the body's immune system.

So, if you are going to snack, be aware that good things don't always come in small packages. Along with calories, you can get a lot of sodium, saturated fat, and other things that you don't want— namely, artificial colors and assorted unappetizing additives.

72. There's Nothing Bright About Artificial Colors

Artificial coal tar–based (azo) dyes have been used extensively as colorings in snack foods and confections for years, though not without objection. Seventeen have finally been banned, delisted, and deemed hazardous by the FDA, but a tenacious seven—FD&C Red No. 3, Blue No. 1, Blue No. 2, Green No. 3, Yellow No. 5, Yellow No. 6, and Red No. 40—remain.

Four of these have been shown to cause cancer and brain tumors in laboratory animals.

Three are under investigation for safety because of assorted toxic findings in research studies.

All are still being used to color our foods.

SOME DYE-HARD SNACKS TO THINK ABOUT

Fruit drops, fruit Jell-O, Kool-Aid, caramels, Lifesavers, fruit drinks, filled chocolates (not pure chocolates), most flavored ice cream, Maraschino cherries, fruit-flavored Popsicles, flavored sodas, pie fillings, "penny" candies, many fruit yogurts, caramel custard, puddings (vanilla, butterscotch, and chocolate), crackers, cheese puffs, virtually all artificially colored candies.

If you are allergic to aspirin, asthmatic, or suffer from exzema, be forewarned that foods containing azo dyes are more likely to affect you adversely.

SOME UNCOLORFUL SIDE EFFECTS

Asthma attacks, hives, watering eye, runny nose, blurred vision, swelling of the skin with fluid, reduction in blood-clotting platelets, hyperactivity in children.

73. Assorted Unappetizing Snack Additives

CARRAGEENAN

A suspected carcinogen, possibly a factor in ulcerative colitis. Most harmful when taken in a beverage. Frequently used in chocolate products (including some chocolate milk), pressure-dispensed whipped cream, cheese spreads, cheese foods, ice cream, frozen custard, sherbets, ices, jellies, and jams.

DEXTRANS

A suspected carcinogen. Most often used in soft-centered candies.

XYLITOL

A suspected carcinogen. Often used in sugarless chewing gums (see section 66).

HYDROGENATED/PARTIALLY HYDROGENATED COCONUT, PALM KERNEL, OR RAPESEED OIL

Highly saturated fats. Used in candy bars, malted milk balls, fruit chews, cookies, crackers, baked confections, whipped toppings, and fruit punches.

MODIFIED FOOD STARCH

A possible health hazard because of the lack of long-term feeding studies; may be a factor in calcium deposits in kidneys and growth retardation. Type of starch used is rarely identified. Used in crackers, cookies, muffins, candies, marshmallows, and fruit punches.

CONFECTIONER'S GLAZE

Refined shellac, made for food use by bleaching regular shellac that's used on furniture. No long-term feeding studies on safety have been done. Used as a coating for many candies and baked confections.

See section 22 for acacia gum, alginates, BHA, BHT, propyl gallate, and others.

74. Smarter Snack Trade-offs

INSTEAD OF...
Potato chips or pretzels, both of which are veritable mines of salt (pretzels have 495 mg. per ounce) and can deplete you of B vitamins, while offering you no nutritional benefits and taxing your liver unfairly.

HOW ABOUT...
Popcorn. It is filling instead of fattening (only 41 calories per ounce), a great source of fiber, and if you sprinkle it with some debittered yeast (not brewer's yeast) instead of salt, you'll have a terrific snack with nutrients galore.

INSTEAD OF...
Salted peanuts, which are roasted in oil and high in fat, sodium, and calories.

HOW ABOUT...
Shelled or unshelled dry unsalted roasted peanuts. You eliminate the sodium and still benefit from protein and B vitamins. Raw peanuts should be cooked quickly at a high temperature (in the oven or a non-stick pan) before eating. This destroys a substance in them that can otherwise interfere with the body's ability to metabolize essential nutrients.

INSTEAD OF...
Packed tortilla chips, such as Doritos, which are made with the most saturated of hydrogenated oils (coconut, palm, and cottonseed) and contain 7 g. of fat per ounce, along with a roster of unwanted additives, including MSG, FD&C Yellow No. 5, and gum arabic, and can turn snack time to allergy attack time.

HOW ABOUT...
Homemade tortilla wedges. Stack five 8-inch flour tortillas and cut into 8 wedges to make 40. Spread these in a single layer on two baking sheets, bake for 10 to 15 minutes at 375°, or until crispy. Instead of 7 g. of fat, you'll get only one—and no unnecessary additive side effects.

INSTEAD OF...
Chocolate, which has numerous strikes against it. (See section 69.)

HOW ABOUT...
Carob, the powered seed of the carob tree. It has a flavor similar to chocolate but contains no theobromine or caffeine—and is much lower in fat.

INSTEAD OF . . .
Ice cream, which is often filled with hidden and potentially harmful additives (see section 22) and has more fat than you need.

How ABOUT . . .
Low-fat yogurt sweetened with fresh fruit or a bit of honey; frozen sherbet; frozen juices made into additive-free Popsicles.

INSTEAD OF . . .
Non-nutritive, chewy caramel candies, which are usually filled with additives and are being investigated by the FDA for nitrogen-containing impurities that might be present in caramel manufactured by an ammonia process.

Go FOR . . .
Dried fruits. (See "Cautions" in section 126.) They are as sweet as candy and good sources of vitamin A (ten dried apricot halves supply more than 3,000 IU) and calcium (raisins have 18 mg. per ounce).

INSTEAD OF . . .
A hot dog or hamburger, both of which have numerous nutritional drawbacks. (See sections 58 & 61.)

Go FOR . . .
A taco or a slice of pizza. These can offer more in the way of vitamins, minerals, and complex carbohydrates and less in the way of fat.

INSTEAD OF . . .
Fast-food shakes, with their high fat and additive content.

Go FOR . . .
Homemade shakes. (Fruit plus ¾ cup powdered milk, ½ cup orange juice, and 1½ cups water with a few ice cubes makes a shake that can be kept cold in a thermos, or frozen and eaten as a Popsicle.)

INSTEAD OF . . .
Chewing gum, which aside from containing empty calories, unwanted additives, and artificial colors and flavorings, stimulates the saliva that prepares the digestive tract for food it doesn't receive, as well as creating increased hunger and gastrointestinal problems.

Go FOR . . .
Raw carrots and celery chips. These satisfy your urge to chew and provide wholesome, health-promoting vitamins and minerals, particularly vitamins A, C, calcium, phosphorus, and potassium, and many essential amino acids.

INSTEAD OF ...	GO FOR ...
Sweets of any kind.	Sunflower seeds. These can actually suppress your urge for sweets (as well as cigarettes, by the way). They release glucose from the liver which then rushes to the brain like adrenaline and produces a similar "lift" effect. The calories are still there (406 in ½ cup), but they offer plenty of protein (17.4 g.), no cholesterol, 5.2 mg. of iron, and a good 87 mg. of calcium.

75. Any Questions About Chapter 6?

I've recently started a diet, and to curb my appetite, I have taken to chewing gum. But I've noticed that after chewing, the blood vessels in my face seem to become redder. Have you any idea why?

I would suspect that the gum contains BHT (see section 22), which frequently causes allergic reactions. Try not chewing gum for a day and keep away from all products containing BHT. If your facial redness doesn't disappear, consult your doctor immediately.

I've read that manufacturers are not required to list all the additives in ice cream because it's a standardized food. Are any of the additives in it harmful, and is there any way then for me to find out which ice creams have the least amount?

All additives are *potentially* harmful. As a rule, the cheaper brands use more synthetic ingredients than the more expensive brands. Those containing piperonal, often used as a substitute for vanilla (as well as a chemical to kill lice); ethyl vanillin, which has caused liver, kidney, heart, lung, and spleen damage in laboratory animals; butyraldehyde, which gives a nutlike flavor to ice cream (and is also an ingredient in rubber cement); and isoamyl acetate, a banana-pear flavor used in many ice creams (and several shoe polishes), are ones I would strongly suggest you avoid.

If you're going to eat ice cream, I would recommend making it yourself (home ice cream makers are relatively inexpensive and you can control the ingredients). If not, buy the better-quality brands. An ice cream with few additives should melt slowly to form a custardlike cream, not a watery liquid. To test, put the edge of a spoon into softened ice cream. When you pull it out, the ice cream should stick to the spoon. If the spoon comes out clean, the ice cream contains more additives than you want.

I have heard of a natural sweetener called amasake. What is it, and is it safe?

Amasake is similar to malt syrups, but it is made from cooked rice, barley, or other grain, and inoculated with *Aspergillus oryzae* mold (koji), which turns grain starch into sugar. Since *Aspergillus* is a fungus source suspected of producing carcinogens during metabolism, I'd say it is a risky sweetener at best and recommend avoiding it. Use honey instead.

7

THINK BEFORE YOU DRINK— ANYTHING

76. Rubbing In the Hard Facts About Alcohol

"Bottoms up!" can be a downer for more people in more ways than they realize.

• Alcohol is not a stimulant, but a sedative-depressant of the central nervous system.

• It can suppress immune system functions, increasing the risk of infection and susceptibility to disease.

• It interferes with proper nutrient absorption.

• It can alter enzymes that normally detoxify carcinogens.

• It is a teratogenic drug. (Pregnant women who drink endanger their unborn children with Fetal Alcohol Syndrome, which can cause, aside from low birth weight, brain damage and physical malformation.)

• It depletes the body of B vitamins (especially folic acid) as well as substantial amounts of calcium, magnesium, zinc, and other trace minerals, all of which are essential emotion energizers.

• It impedes the formation and storage of glycogen in the liver; in other words, it reduces your fitness fuel.

• It impairs coordination and reduces the contractile strength of muscles.

• It worsens allergic reactions to foods.

• It is capable of rupturing veins.

• Its dehydrating properties (which cause morning-after thirst) can destroy brain cells by withdrawing necessary water from them.

• Chronic use can cause memory lapses, impaired learning ability, motor disturbances, and general disorientation.

• Over one million Americans are allergic to ingredients in alcoholic beverages that can cause severe adverse reactions.

• Four drinks a day are capable of causing organ damage.

• Anyone who has acquired a tolerance to alcohol might need larger doses of sedatives or tranquilizers to be effective. This hazardous combination increases the possibility of an unwitting overdose.

• Alcohol can interact adversely with more than one hundred medications, with effects ranging from simple nausea to sudden death.

CAUTION: Unless you have asked and been told by your physician that you can have a drink with another drug, DON'T!

77. Beer Is Nothing to Cheer About

It's touted as the ultimate reward for a hard day's work—winning ball games, getting together with friends, and celebrating jobs well done—but that doesn't mean that beer is something to cheer about.

Though the alcohol in a 12-ounce can of beer is just as intoxicating as the alcohol in a 5-ounce glass of wine and a 1½ ounce shot of 80 proof liquor (and no less harmful), beer labels don't even have to indicate that beer is an alcoholic beverage. Furthermore, beer contains more than just barley water, malt, hops, and yeast. A lot more.

BEER ADDITIVES THAT BREW TROUBLE

• *Aspergillus oryzae,* a fungus source suspected of producing a carcinogen during metabolism.

• Papain, shown to be an antigen which, besides causing a specific allergic response, can enlarge ranges of sensitivity.

• Acacia (gum arabic), a foam stabilizer gushing with drawbacks (see section 22).

• Alginate (propylene glycol alginate), which has been shown to cause fetal and maternal deaths in laboratory animals and is considered a health risk for pregnant women.

• Calcium disodium EDTA, which can cause gastrointestinal upsets and kidney damage, and is still being investigated by the UN Joint FAO/WHO Expert Committee on Food Additives for possible mutagenic, teratogenic, and reproductive effects. (NOTE: EDTA has blood-thinning properties that might affect dosage levels if you are taking anticoagulant medication.)

• Sulfites galore (potassium metabisulfite, sodium bisulfite, sodium hydrosulfite, sodium metabisulfite) used as antioxidants and potentially dangerous for many people. (See section 26.)

• Artificial colors, including FD&C Blue No. 1, Red No. 40, and Yellow No. 5. (See section 72.)

• Nitrosamines (see section 35), unintentionally formed when malted barley is dried by direct firing, but nonetheless carcinogenic. (The U.S. brewing industry has modified its barley-drying process and reduced nitrosamine levels, but nitrosamines at any level are still nitrosamines.)

78. The Heavy Truth About Light Beers

No matter how you spell it (light or lite), low-calorie beers aren't weight reducers.

A 12-ounce glass of light beer that should contain approximately 98 calories, or one-third the calories of regular beer (approximately 150 calories), sometimes has about as many calories as regular beer. Michelob Light, for example, has 135 calories—only 5 calories less than regular Coors, and only 1 calorie less than Hamm's. And if you are dieting, 50 fewer calories a glass is about as significant as not eating 5 potato chips—which, if you're a beer drinker, you will probably eat anyway.

Light beers do have less alcohol than regular brews, but not enough to deem them safe for indiscriminate consumption by pregnant women, or anyone with a sulfite sensitivity. Also, because there is no legal definition of "light," the "light" on a beer label might simply be used to distinguish a paler brew from a darker one.

79. Nonalcoholic Trade-offs Pay Off

For drinkers who enjoy the taste of malt and hops, but don't want the calories or consequences of alcohol, nonalcoholic beers are probably the best trade-offs around.

Compared with an average of 150 calories in 12 ounces of regular beer, nonalcoholic beer contains about 50 calories. And as far as alcohol goes, you would have to drink about a hundred bottles of nonalcoholic beer on the wall to come close to consuming 6 ounces.

Nonalcoholic beer, by law, can contain only trace amounts of alcohol (½ percent by volume), which is less than what you get in a tablespoon of most over-the-counter cough and cold medicines. (NOTE: Products that are labeled "alcohol free" cannot contain *any* alcohol.)

CAUTION: Nonalcoholic beer is contraindicated for alcoholics.

80. The Grapes of Wrath

Whoever said *"In vino veritas"* wasn't talking about truth in wine labeling. Despite being one of the most cherished beverages around the world, most people know little more about wine than that it is fermented grape juice (or in the case of sake, a Japanese wine, fermented rice).

Wine lovers will argue that labels tell a lot. They give such important information as where the wine comes from, who produced it, and when and where it was bottled. A label that doesn't give the name of the vineyard where the grapes were grown indicates that the wine may be a blend of wines, usually of inferior taste, since the good wines in a blend are used to upgrade the mediocre ones. A label without a vintage year also indicates a blend of wines from different years. (In California it is legal to add 5 percent of wine from another year to any vintage bottle.) Wine labels will also list the name of the importer and the alcohol content by volume, which can vary from 8.5 percent (a few French and German wines) to 21 percent (sherry and port); American wines generally have an alcohol content of 12 to 14 percent.

But wine labels don't tell you what else you are getting. For example, sulfur dioxide or potassium metabisulfite (which are used to kill bacteria on grapes, or stop yeast action when fermentation has reached the desired point), both of which can seriously endanger sulfite-sensitive individuals (see section 26).

Other chemicals used in wine-making that are potential health hazards for many people are:

- Acacia (gum arabic)
- Albumen (egg white)
- Antifoaming and defoaming agents, such as polyoxyethylene-40-monostearate and silicon dioxide
- Casein, potassium salt of casein, and milk powder
- Copper sulfate
- Ferrocyanide compounds
- Lactic and malic acids
- Mineral oil
- Proplyene glycol

The following list, based on tests commissioned by the Center for Science in the Public Interest (CSPI), gives the approximate sulphur dioxide content of some popular wines to help allergy-prone wine lovers make trade-offs that could minimize adverse reactions.

WINE	SULFUR DIOXIDE PER 750 ML. BOTTLE
Almaden	
Calif. French Colombard	125 mg.
Mountain Red Burgundy	104 mg.
Cella	
Rosato	100 mg.
Lambrusco	87 mg.
Christian Brothers	
Calif. Chablis	81 mg.
Select Calif. Burgundy	42 mg.
Gallo	
Chablis Blanc	111 mg.
Hearty Burgundy	74 mg.

WINE	SULFUR DIOXIDE PER 750 ML. BOTTLE
Giacobazzi	
Bianco	122 mg.
Lambrusco	80 mg.
Inglenook	
Navalle Chablis	102 mg.
Navalle Zinfandel	87 mg.
Paul Masson	
Calif. French Colombard	133 mg.
Calif. Chablis	145 mg.
Calif. Burgundy	78 mg.
Emerald Dry	160 mg.
Riunite	
Rosato	67 mg.
Bianco	55 mg.
Lambrusco	80 mg.
Sebastiani	
Calif. Mountain Chablis	188 mg.
Calif. Mountain Red Burgundy	48 mg.
Taylor California Cellars	
Chenin Blanc	89 mg.
Zinfandel	52 mg.

At this time the government permits wine-makers to use over eighty additives. All are certainly not used in any one wine, and many are removed before bottling, but if you have any questions about what's in the wine you are drinking I would suggest you write to the wineries. Their addresses are usually on the labels. If not, your local wine merchant can probably get them for you.

81. Why Wine Coolers Are Not So Hot

They look like soft drinks, but they are half alcohol (6 percent by volume) and half fruit juice, and contain more sugar than almost any other beverage around (which is probably why the calorie content is conspicuously omitted from virtually all their labels).

The majority of brands boast that they're made with "natural" fruit juice, and that they contain "no artificial flavors." But a close look at labels reveals that these contain artificial colors, along with sulfur dioxide, potassium sorbate, and sodium benzoate, all of which can cause a wide variety of allergic reactions (see section 24), and added sugar.

CAUTION: These are alcoholic beverages and should be kept out of the reach of children, who can easily mistake them for soft drinks. They are also contraindicated for alcoholics, or anyone taking any medications, *particularly* antidepressants, barbiturates, painkillers, and disulfiram (Antabus).

82. Liquor Facts That Won't Raise Your Spirits

If you are a drinker, the good news is that 80 to 100 proof whiskeys contain sufficient alcohol (40 to 50 percent) to destroy bacteria, control yeast, and eliminate the need for antifoaming agents. So except for a little ethylenediaminetetraacetate, which is used in brewing (though under investigation for harmful effects), and some questionably safe caramel coloring, most hard liquors are relatively additive free. The bad news is that there are no labels to tell you which ones aren't.

If you're a Scotch drinker, there is more bad news. Because of the way malted barley is dried, Scotch has been found to contain small amounts of carcinogenic nitrosamines.

And there's even more bad news if you are into liqueurs or premixed cocktails. These contain artificial colorings, flavorings, and synthetic cream bases. There are, of course, some products that use real cream (Bailey's Original Irish Cream liqueur, for instance), but because of its cost, the cream in most "crème" liqueurs is generally non-dairy creamer (see section 51). Check the label before you drink. Alcohol and additives are enough of a nutritional body blow without adding saturated fat.

NOTE: Real cream liqueurs should be kept refrigerated after opening to prevent spoilage.

83. Taking the Fizz Out of Soft Drinks

Not counting the myriad fruit-flavored beverages such as Kool-Aid, Tang, and Hi-C, 21 percent of the sugar in the American diet comes from soft drinks! That's more than just an unhealthy consumption of empty calories. It is a dangerous overload of caffeine (see section 42) and potentially hazardous, nutrient-depleting additives.

HARD FACTS ABOUT SOFT DRINKS

• Soft drinks contain large amounts of phosphorus, which can throw off the body's calcium/phosphorous ratio (twice as much calcium as phosphorus), decreasing calcium as well as reducing your body's ability to use it.

• For anyone over forty, soft drinks can be especially hazardous because the kidneys are less able to excrete excess phosphorus, causing depletion of vital calcium.

• Heavy soft drink consumption can interfere with your body's metabolization of iron and diminish nerve impulse transmission.

• Sodas may contain—but are not required to disclose—such ingredients as ethyl alcohol, sodium alginate (possibly hazardous for pregnant women), brominated vegetable oil (found harmful to vital organs of animals and considered a health risk to heavy consumers of beverages containing it), and caffeine.

• Cola drinks can interact adversely with antacids, possibly causing constipation, calcium loss, hypertension, nausea, vomiting, headaches, and kidney damage.

• Soft drinks can decrease the antibacterial action of penicillin and ampicillin.

• The average 12-ounce cola has 150 calories and over an ounce (7 teaspoons) of refined sugar; a 12-ounce un-cola has 7½ teaspoons of sugar.

• Diet sodas that are low in calories are *high* in sodium. (Six ounces of regular Pepsi-Cola have 5 mg. of sodium; Diet Pepsi has 31 mg.)

NOTE: Salt is just as dangerous to your health as sugar (see section 93), and is sometimes more depressing for dieters who don't understand that it causes the retention of water, which can add pounds despite your subtraction of calories.

84. Unwatered-down Truths About Water

A human being can live for weeks without food, but for only a few days without water. It is our most important nutrient; nothing takes place in our bodies without it.

- It is the best solvent for all the products of digestion.
- It is essential for removing wastes.
- It is indispensable for transporting nutrients, building tissues, and regulating body temperature.
- It has no known toxicity when unadulterated, though an intake of 1½ gallons (16-24 glasses) in about an hour could be dangerous to an adult and kill an infant.
- It is, without question, the elixir of life—and it is poisoning millions of us daily.

If you have never given much thought to the water you've been drinking, you could be in trouble. Water contamination is here and it's on the rise. (The Environmental Protection Agency has a priority list of approximately 129 dangerous water pollutants.) Pesticides, hazardous waste dumps, and industrial dumping of untreated garbage into rivers and landfills, as well as chemical additives used in the treatment of drinking water, are just some of the contributors to the increasing pollution of our drinking water.

How dangerous are these contaminants? Well, solvent chemicals, such as polychlorinated biphenyls (PCBs) and chloroform, are suspected carcinogens. Others have been found to cause central nervous system disorders and reproductive problems.

Tap water with the wrong PH (due to improper water treatment of acid rain) can dissolve lead from pipes, subjecting young children to lead poisoning, which can cause mental retardation. People living in older homes containing lead pipes should definitely have their water analyzed by their local county health department. In fact, even homes with copper plumbing can have lead-soldered joints that might affect tap water.

85. How Safe Is Your Tap Water?

The following table, based on an EPA study of drinking water purified for human consumption in major U.S. cities, shows the levels of suspected carcinogenic substances still present.

CARCINOGENS ON TAP

Albuquerque, NM	15 mcg.
Atlanta, GA	75 mcg.
Baltimore, MD	65 mcg.
Birmingham, AL	75 mcg.
Boise, ID	16 mcg.
Boston, MA	5 mcg.
Buffalo, NY	23 mcg.
Casper, WY	41 mcg.
Charleston, SC	200 mcg.
Chicago, IL	50 mcg.
Cleveland, OH	49 mcg.
Dallas, TX	79 mcg.
Denver, CO	39 mcg.
Des Moines, IA	15 mcg.
Detroit, MI	34 mcg.
Fresno, CA	4 mcg.
Grand Rapids, MI	69 mcg.
Hartford, CT	36 mcg.
Houston, TX	250 mcg.
Indianapolis, IN	82 mcg.
Kansas City, KS	34 mcg.
Las Vegas, NV	76 mcg.
Little Rock, AR	42 mcg.
Los Angeles, CA	49 mcg.
Louisville, KY	150 mcg.
Memphis, TN	17 mcg.
Milwaukee, WI	16 mcg.
Minneapolis, MN	90 mcg.
Nashville, TN	24 mcg.
Oklahoma City, OK	200 mcg.
Omaha, NE	120 mcg.

CARCINOGENS ON TAP

Phoenix, AZ	130 mcg.
Pittsburgh, PA	43 mcg.
Portland, ME	7 mcg.
Providence, RI	8 mcg.
Tampa, FL	230 mcg.
Salt Lake City, UT	43 mcg.
San Antonio, TX	13 mcg.
San Diego, CA	97 mcg.
San Francisco, CA	78 mcg.
Sioux Falls, SD	79 mcg.
St. Louis, MO	51 mcg.
Tulsa, OK	50 mcg.
Washington, DC	110 mcg.
Wichita, KS	27 mcg.

86. The Hazards of Home Water Filters

More and more people are being solicited by water filtering companies, which come to your home, test your water, and frighten you enough to sign up for an installation of their product right on the spot.

There are different systems used for processing water that comes from your public supply center, and you should be aware of the drawbacks of all of them.

THE REVERSE-OSMOSIS SYSTEM

Reverse osmosis (RO) has been used for years by industries for large-scale removal of salt from seawater to produce drinking water. Home RO systems remove not only salts, but also sediments and other minerals, cleansing water of chemicals and providing clean, clear taste.

A good system will have a sediment prefilter as well as a carbon filter, because most of the water that goes into an RO module comes out again as wastewater, or brine. It will remove a large range of chemicals, but it is not that effective in processing inorganic contaminants. *RO product water must be tested periodicallly to monitor the performance of the system*. A filter may be able to eliminate the large molecules that add tastes and odors long after it has lost the ability to remove small organic contaminants (chloroform, for instance). And all filters may lose their chemical-removing capacity long before your water flow becomes sluggish.

CAUTION: A filter can also be loaded with bacteria and not show a reduced flow rate.

ACTIVATED CARBON FILTERS

These remove undissolved metals such as iron, lead, manganese, and copper, and are best for removing organic chemicals, which is their prime value. They do not remove magnesium or calcium; water softeners are needed for that.

CAUTION: Water softeners add sodium to the water, which can unhealthily increase your daily salt intake.

An activated carbon filter will also trap some low-level bacteria that are present in all purified water. But if the filter is left unused for any length of time, these small amounts of bacteria can multiply into potentially harmful numbers.

Activated carbon filters that are not changed on a regular basis can become fouled with harmful contaminants. Also, avoid units containing silver as a bacteriostat. Silver has not been shown to be an effective bacteria killer and can be harmful in itself if it leaches into your drinking water.

DISTILLERS

These heat water to the boiling point in a chamber. Contaminated liquids remain trapped in the chamber, while other liquids that boil at lower temperatures are vented off as vapors. The steam is then cooled until it condenses into a purified state, when it is collected in a storage reservoir until ready for use.

A distiller is not as effective in removing organic contaminants as it is in removing inorganic dissolved solids. (Using an activated charcoal filter with a distiller will increase its organic-removal rate to over 90 percent.) Distillers also require electricity for their heating elements, and when in operation they produce a large amount of heat (often enough to heat a small room), which may or may not be desirable, depending on its location and the time of year.

CAUTION: A distiller must be descaled regularly. If instructions aren't followed carefully, the product water can be worse instead of better.

87. Bottled Alternatives

Just because water is sold in a bottle doesn't mean that it is pure. All water, except distilled, is mineral water and contains impurities (though not necessarily harmful ones).

MINERAL WATER CONFUSION

Minerals in water are measured by a lump measurement known as "total dissolved solids" (TDS). Because of a California-initiated regulation (the FDA has not officially defined "mineral water"), if a bottled water has 500 ppm (parts per million) or more of TDS, it must be labeled "mineral water," even if the minerals themselves have little to do with the water's quality. On the other hand, if the water has less than 500 ppm it cannot be labeled a mineral water.

This has caused confusion for consumers and consternation for bottlers. Perrier just barely made it as a mineral water with 545 ppm TDS. Poland Spring, which has been calling itself a mineral water for more than seventy years, is too pure (less than 126 ppm TDS for both their still and sparkling waters) and had to change its label. And Canada Dry Club Soda had to plead for an exemption to keep its well-recognized label, when it was discovered that the beverage contains 536 ppm TDS.

Some bottled "mineral waters" may actually have fewer dissolved minerals than many city water supplies. In fact, the term "mineral water" is frequently used to describe all bottled water, with the exception of bulk water, club soda, and seltzer.

"Natural" mineral water, sparkling or still, usually comes from a spring and contains only the minerals present in the water as it flows from the ground. Mineral water without the word "natural" on its label may have had minerals removed or added. Calistoga Water, for example, comes from a geyser in California's Napa Valley, where the mineral content is high, and therefore minerals are removed; Schweppes and Calso, both formulated from tap water, add minerals.

CAUTION: If you're watching your sodium intake, watch out for Calso Mineral Water. One 8-ounce glass contains an incredible 397 mg. of sodium—more than anyone needs in a day.

TAPPING INTO SPRING WATER

All "spring water" must, under truth-in-labeling laws, come from a spring (Deer Park 100% Spring Water, Evian Natural Spring Water). It may already be carbonated, as is the case with Vittelloise Natural Spring Water, or add carbonation, which is what Deer Park Sparkling 100% Spring Water does.

The word "natural" implies that the water has not been processed in any way before bottling, whereas plain "spring water" may or may not go right into the bottle. Anything simply labeled "drinking water" generally comes from a well or the tap, and is usually processed before bottling.

Bulk waters are usually purified tap water. The word "spring" is often cleverly used as part of a company's name so that it appears to be a description of their product, which it is not.

STILL VERSUS SPARKLING

Still water has no gas bubbles. Sparkling water is made bubbly by dissolved carbon dioxide gas, which can occur naturally in subsurface water or added later. (The gas in most "naturally sparkling" waters, such as Perrier and Saratoga, is drawn off at the spring and reinjected during bottling.) Still water can be carbonated with either natural carbon dioxide (Poland Spring Sparkling fizzes its Maine water with carbon dioxide mined in Colorado) or manufactured carbon dioxide, which is what Canada Dry Club Soda uses.

The difference? Natural carbon dioxide usually produces longer-lasting bubbles.

CLUB SODA AND SELTZER

If you want carbonated water with no added frills (minerals or mineral salts) go for seltzer. It is filtered, carbonated tab water, period. Club soda is also filtered, carbonated tap water, but minerals and mineral salts are added. If you are trying to cut down on your sodium, choose seltzer. Six ounces of Schweppes Club Soda have 26 mg. of salt.

88. Any Questions About Chapter 7?

A landfill has just been built about a mile from where I live, and I am worried about my well water being contaminated. A company in my area tests water, but I've heard that it tells everyone something is wrong with the water just to sell its purifiers. Is there any way I can test my own water?

Yes, there is. Water Test (see section 145) does analyses nationwide by mail order. It provides a basic test package that gives you a screening for about $100. But I would advise that you first speak to your local health officials and find out about the kinds of contaminants you should look for. The most common are coliform bacteria, nitrates and nitrites, trace metals, toxic chemicals, and trihalomethanes (though these are unlikely to be in well water since they are formed by chlorine reacting with other substances).

Meanwhile, until you are sure that your water is safe, you should take the following emergency measures:

• Let your water run for 3 to 4 minutes every day before using it. This will help flush out any lead, cadmium, and cobalt that may be lodging in your pipes.

• Boil your water (uncovered) for at least 20 minutes before using it. Boiling can kill bacteria and remove some organic chemicals.

• If you are worried about trihalomethanes, whip your water in a blender for 15 minutes with the top off. Aeration removes chlorine and chlorinated organics.

CAUTION: If you suspect that chlorinated solvents or pesticides are in your water, be aware that these chemicals can be absorbed through the skin and are volatile. *Taking one 15-minute shower can be as toxic as drinking 8 glasses of contaminated water.*

My seven-year-old son frequently swallows mouthwash instead of spitting it out. Is there any real danger in this?

A very real danger. Most brands of mouthwash contain substantial amounts of alcohol, as much as 15 to 29 percent. (To give you some perspective, beer has only 5 to 7 percent, and wine about 12 to 14 percent.) The fact that your son likes the taste increases the risk of his drinking it when you're not around, which could have disastrous results. Even small amounts can affect your son's central nervous system, causing decreased reaction time, muscular incoordination, and behavioral changes, as well as interfere with any medications he might be taking. Also, incidences of poisoning through accidental ingestion of mouthwashes by children have become all too common.

Equally frightening is that there may be a relationship between mouthwash usage and oral cancers. According to research done by Dr. Stephen Z. Wolner, D.D.S., regular use of mouthwash puts consumers at high risk for the development of malignant oral cancers. While all the evidence is not yet in, there is enough to warrant playing it safe. In fact, an FDA advisory committee has already declared that antibacterial agents are not necessary to freshen the mouth, that there is no evidence that mouthwash "germ-killing" agents are effective, and that they might even retard healing!

I would strongly advise you to keep mouthwash out of your son's mouth as well as his reach. Brushing and flossing regularly are far better for his teeth and health (as well as yours), and water is a fine, efficient rinse.

Why is it that some alcoholic drinks give me a hangover while others don't?

Distilled spirits have varying amounts of substances known as congeners. They are the result of fermentation and maturation of liquor and contribute to its flavor. They also cause hangovers. Whereas alcohol can be eliminated fairly rapidly from the body, congeners cannot.

There are different types and amounts of congeners in drinks, and their adverse effects depend on your sensitivity to them. Some people can knock back six shots of vodka without blinking an eye, but give them a jigger of bourbon and they are looped. For others, it could be just the opposite.

As a rule, though, the more congeners a beverage has, the more splitting the hangover. Vodka and gin have the least congeners; bourbon has the most. Nonetheless, brandy seems to produce the majority of hangovers, followed in morning-after infamy by red wine (which has substances very similar to congeners), rum, whiskey, white wine, gin, and vodka.

I read recently that some German and Italian imported wines were found to contain a toxic chemical. Do you know what it is? If so, could you tell me how dangerous it is? I drink a lot of imported wines, and I am quite concerned.

I can't blame you. The chemical is diethylene glycol, a component in antifreeze. It was present in only small amounts in the wines, but it does have cumulative toxic effects in the body. The wines to keep away from are:

• 1984 Haus Franz Liebfraumilch and 1984 Haus Frickenstein Liebfraumilch, both Qualitätswein A.P. 1 907 021 29 84
• 1984 Haus Franz Liebfraumilch Rheinpfalz Qualitätswein A.P. 5 907 021 518 84
• 1982 Wolfsheimer Abtey Kabinett A.P. 4 907 183 109 84
• 1983 Saulheimer Domherr Eiswein A.P. 4 907 183 108 84
• 1981 Barbera D'Asti; 1980 Barbaresco; 1973 Gattinara; Non-vintage Asti Spumante; 1981 D'Aquino Barbera D'Asti. Bottled by F. Li Dogliani, La Morra, Italy
• 1979 Kiola Barola, bottled by FDO, La Morra, Italy
• Non-vintage Lambrusco, bottled by Stapis, Calmasino, Italy
• 1980 Kiola Barbaresco, bottled by FDO, La Morra, Italy

8

FOR WHOM THE DINNER BELLS TOLL

89. The Big Supper Mistake

For most people, dinner is the largest meal of the day, and it shouldn't be.

• It's the time when we need the least number of calories, yet consume the most.
• It's the time when we consume the most amount of protein, fat, carbohydrates, and sodium, but need them the least.
• It's the meal we feel makes up for skipped breakfasts and poor lunches, but it doesn't.
• It's the most misunderstood, mishandled meal of the day.

Before sitting down for dinner it is important to consider what else you've eaten that day. Ignoring the fact that you had a croissant for breakfast and a hamburger with fries for lunch can be risky if you're planning to have a full-course steak dinner. It can take you well over your recommended limit of daily fat, protein, sodium and calories, and trip you up in innumerable nutritional ways. The following guide has been designed to help prevent this from happening.

HEALTHY AMOUNTS FOR HEALTHIER LIVING

CALORIES AND FAT

AGE	RECOMMENDED DAILY CALORIE INTAKE	RECOMMENDED DAILY FAT INTAKE	
(children) 1–3	1,300	8 tsp.	35.2 g.
4–6	1,700	11 tsp.	48.4 g.
7–10	2,400	15 tsp.	66.0 g.
(males) 11–14	2,700	17 tsp.	74.8 g.
15–18	2,800	18 tsp.	79.2 g.
19–22	2,900	18 tsp.	79.2 g.
23–50	2,700	17 tsp.	74.8 g.
51–74	2,400	15 tsp.	66.0 g.
75+	2,050		
(females) 11–14	2,220	14 tsp.	61.6 g.
15–22	2,100	13 tsp.	57.2 g.
23–50	2,000	13 tsp.	57.2 g.
51–74	1,800	11 tsp.	48.4 g.
75+	1,600		

PROTEIN AND SODIUM

AGE	RECOMMENDED DAILY PROTEIN INTAKE IN G.	RECOMMENDED DAILY SODIUM INTAKE IN MG.
(children) 1–3	23 g.	650 mg.
4–6	30 g.	900 mg.
7–10	34 g.	1,200 mg.
(males) 11–14	45 g.	1,800 mg.
15–18	56 g.	1,800 mg.
19–74+	56 g.	2,220 mg.
(females) 11–18	46 g.	1,800 mg.
19–74+	44 g.	2,200 mg.

90. Meaty Problems

We eat too much meat for our own good. Just half a pound of lean ground beef supplies all of a woman's daily requirement for protein; three-quarters of a pound has more than what is recommended for a man.

There is no question that meat is an excellent source of protein, and that protein is the major source of building material for the body, but eating too much of it can be hazardous to your health (see section 91). And eating too much in the form of animal flesh can be even more hazardous.

> You could be getting your steak with a hidden side order of drugs.

Aside from meat's potential for supplying us with more protein than we need and more saturated fat than we should have, it is insidiously giving us drugs we don't want. The majority of American livestock is routinely given subtherapeutic doses of antibiotics such as penicillin and tetracycline. Because subtherapeutic doses are smaller than those needed to control an actual infection, they kill off susceptible bacteria and allow resistant ones to thrive, promoting the spread of antibiotic-resistant bacteria—which is being transmitted to humans!

The alarming increase of antibiotic-resistant bacteria in humans has caused numerous outbreaks of gastrointestinal infections, as well as eighteen documented cases of antibiotic-resistant salmonellosis (one fatal) caused by the consumption of hamburger from cattle that had been treated with chlortetracycline as a growth promoter.

The presence of these drug residues poses enormous health risks for everyone.

• A person allergic to penicillin, for instance, could suffer the same adverse reaction by eating a roast beef sandwich if the animal the beef came from had been dosed with that drug.

• Antibiotics that have been used successfully to treat numerous illnesses and infections are being rendered ineffective because of our increasing acquisition of antibiotic-resistant bacteria. (Already, 20 percent of the organisms responsible for strep throat can no longer be killed by tetracycline, and 25 percent of influenza bacteria are unaffected by penicillin.)

• Many chemicals being used (albeit illegally) in animal feed are known carcinogens.

Unfortunately, there is no way to tell if your meat (or chicken, eggs, and milk) is tainted with drug residues. But you can minimize the risk to yourself and family in several ways.

• Eat fewer animal products.
• Have your steaks and burgers well done.
• Find out where to buy meats, poultry, and eggs that come from animals raised without drugs. The USDA's Food Safety and Inspection Service (see section 145) may be able to help.

91. Resolving the Protein Predicament

Everyone knows that protein is essential for life. It is vital for the growth, development and repair of all body tissues, the regulation of the body's water balance, the formation of hormones and enzymes necessary for basic life functions, antibodies needed to fight infection, and more. But too much of a good thing can be bad for you.

THE PROBLEMS OF TOO MUCH PROTEIN

• It can shorten life expectancy.
• It can increase the risk of cancer and heart disease.
• It can stress and damage the liver and kidneys.
• It can deplete calcium from bones and promote osteoporosis.
• It can cause fluid imbalance and dehydration.
• It can be hazardous to premature infants.
• It can contribute significantly to obesity.
• It increases your need for vitamin B_6.

Excessive protein consumption is generally the result of diets overloaded with meat, cheese, poultry, eggs, and fish, and under-supplied with legumes, grains, and vegetables.

Meat, cheese, poultry, eggs, and fish are *complete proteins*. They provide the proper balance of all the essential amino acids (those that cannot, like others, be manufactured by the human body and must be obtained from food or supplements), and are widely—but erroneously—believed to be (a) healthier, (b) nonfattening, and (c) harmless when eaten in large amounts.

Legumes, grains, and vegetables are *incomplete proteins*. They lack certain essential amino acids and are not used efficiently when eaten alone, which might account for their being widely—but erroneously—believed to be (a) optional, (b) fattening, and (c) wholesome when eaten in small amounts.

PUTTING PROTEIN IN PERSPECTIVE

• Complete proteins generally have more fat than protein.
• Incomplete proteins combined with rice, corn, or grains can become wholesome, low-fat complete proteins.
• *Mixing complete and incomplete proteins can give you better nutrition than having either one alone!*

92. Why Not a Low-fat Chicken in Every Pot?

The same poultry industry that adulterated their feed to breed chickens bigger, fatter, and faster is now feeding their birds low-calorie, high-protein food (ingredients unknown) to reduce their fat and increase their price. The result is chickens that have approximately 14-21% less fat.

Everyone knows that less fat is better. What they don't know is that as impressive as a 14-21% reduction sounds, it's less than 2 grams of fat for an average 4.6 ounce serving, which is the amount of fat in half a pat (½ teaspoon) of butter. Not very impressive. What makes it even less impressive is that fat reductions vary enormously from brand to brand, and have been found to be even wider within a particular brand.

Chicken has always been lower in fat and cholesterol than meat, and the major component of its taste is bound in its fat. As long as low-fat chickens have erratic and dubious fat reductions, you're better off defatting your own.

For whole roasters or broilers: Remove the yellow fat globules that are just inside the cavity near the tail. (They can usually be pulled out with your fingers, but a paring knife will ensure success.)

For chicken parts: Yellow fat globules are visible on the thighs and rib cage. Pull or cut them off.

For significant fat reduction: Remove fat *and skin* before cooking. Skinned chicken should be cooked slowly to prevent unappetizing dryness. Braising in a covered pan with water or broth and vegetables is the best way to retain flavor and nutrients.

When making chicken soup, you can leave skin on while cooking (for flavor), but be sure to skim fat off when the soup is cool. (NOTE: Capons and large hens have more fat than roasters or broilers.)

93. Please Pass on the Salt

You know those two shakers that are on dinner tables? Stay away from the one with the small holes. It's a killer. Asking someone to pass it to you is committing nutritional hari-kari.

High salt consumption can cause hypertension, migraine headaches, abnormal fluid retention, and potassium loss; interfere with proper utilization of protein; increase your chances of heart disease and other serious ailments.

The shaker with the small holes is a killer.

Sodium is in virtually all our foods. The average American consumes about a bowling ball of it (15 pounds) each year. So, if you think you don't eat much salt because you never eat pretzels or chips, you had better think again before dinner.

SNEAKY SUPPER SALT TRAPS

• Tomato juice is a great low-calorie appetizer, but it is high in sodium. Six ounces of Del Monte's have 478 mg.; Campbell's has 555 mg.

• Condiments look harmless, but one 11-calorie dill pickle has 1,426 mg. of sodium.

• Use 2 tablespoons of ketchup on (or in) your meatloaf and you have added 308 mg. of sodium; 2 tablespoons of mustard will give you 444 mg.

• If you are starting with soup, a cup of chicken noodle has 979 mg.; a cup of onion has 1,051 mg.

• A cup of raw celery in your salad and you have 151 mg. sodium; add 2 tablespoons of Italian dressing and you have 624 mg. more.

• Eat a 2-inch square of corn bread with your meal and you have piled on another 283 mg.

• A one-pound lobster has 1,359 mg., and that's without the melted butter, which has 1,120 mg. in half a cup.

• If you want cooked carrots, you'll get only 51 mg. in a cup, if they are fresh; if they are canned, you'll get 366 mg.

• A standard piece of apple pie for dessert has 486 mg.; black coffee, 59 mg.

Put them all together and they spell trouble, with a capital T.

94. Processed Foods That Have Added Nutritional Hazards

When planning a quick 'n easy dinner with processed foods, beware. The FDA's request that the food industry voluntarily reduce salt in their products has been largely ignored. A two-year study of over 185 product lines revealed that sodium was lowered in 29 percent of them, but raised in 26 percent. The following is a list of a few offenders that you might want to keep off your dinner plates.

SOME PRODUCTS THAT HAVE INCREASED THEIR SALT CONTENT

• Armour Dinner Classics frozen dinners
• Chef Boyardee lasagna, pizza, and sauces in jars
• French's seasoning mixes
• Green Giant frozen vegetables

- Kraft Barbecue Sauce and processed cheese
- Progresso soups
- Stouffer frozen soups
- Van de Kamp Mexican and Chinese Classic Entrees
- Weaver poultry products

The Center for Science in the Public Interest (CSPI) cautions consumers not to be fooled by designer boxes of frozen dinners, since these do not have anything to do with nutrition. They also selected the five best on the basis that the product contain less than 700 mg. of sodium, get less than 30 percent of its calories from fat, and provide a minimum of 25 percent of the U.S. RDA for vitamins A and C.

THE CSPI'S TOP FIVE

1. Celentano Cannelloni Florentine
2. Green Giant Sweet & Sour Chicken
3. Legume Tofu Bourgignon
4. Legume Sesame Ginger Stir Fry
5. Light & Elegant Lasagna Florentine

NOTE: When purchasing frozen dinners, buy only those that are frozen solid. Avoid any that feel soft, indicating that they have started to thaw. Refreezing after thawing lowers quality and destroys nutrients.

95. Are You Getting the Full Fish Story?

We have all been told that we should eat more fish—but there's a lot we have *not* been told about some of the fish we're eating.

CATCH-OF-THE-DAY CAUTIONS

Bonito: Sold fresh in supermarkets throughout the country, and canned by both Star-Kist and Pan-Pacific canneries, bonito have been found to contain low levels of DDT and PCBs.

Ocean perch: Those caught in the Pacific Ocean have been found to have relatively high levels of DDT and PCBs.

Pacific mackerel: A California catch that is sold throughout the country and has been found to contain significant levels of DDT.

Red snapper: Rockfish, rock cod, bocaccio and cod, brought in from San Pedro and Newport harbors, have been sold as "red snapper" and found to contain high levels of DDT.

Sablefish: Sometimes known as butterfish, this is frequently sold as cod or sea trout. Those caught off the California coast were found to have only a moderate amount of DDT contaminants, and traces of PCBs.

Swordfish: Those that come from Pacific waters have been found to have low, but potentially hazardous concentrations of PCBs.

White croakers: One of the most abundant species sold in fresh-fish markets on the West Coast, they have the highest concentrations of DDT and PCB contaminants.

HEALTH-RISK POTENTIAL

According to a formula created by the EPA's Carcinogen Assessment Group to assess lifetime health risks associated with the ingestion of carcinogens such as DDT and PCBs (a lifetime risk involves a regular diet of fish over a seventy-year period), eating one half pound of croakers per week could produce 4.4 additional cancers per 10,000 people.

SAFER FISH TRADE-OFFS

- Farm-raised trout
- Alaskan pollack
- Alaskan and Norwegian salmon
- Skipjack and frigate tuna

- Halibut
- Sole
- Turbot

96. What the FDA Has to Say About Your Fish

The FDA limits for acceptable DDT and PCBs in fish are based on the consumption of about 10 g. (⅓ ounce) seafood daily. Their limit of

2 ppm (parts per million) for PCBs in seafood is based on the fact that only 15 percent of fish eaters eat any of the fish that checked in with the highest PCB levels, and those that do consume only one-tenth of an ounce per day.

Now, that's a pretty small amount for any fish eater. So, if you eat more than a 4-ounce serving of a contaminated species more than once every 40 days, it is essentially your problem—which it obviously is.

97. Yes, You Still Should Have Fish for Dinner

Not all fish contain man-made contaminants. In fact, many are not only safe to eat, but also offer enough substantial health benefits for the American Medical Association, the *Journal of the National Cancer Institute,* and virtually all nutritionists to recommend eating them two to four times weekly. The reason is unsaturated fatty acids in fish called Omega-3.

EPA (eicosapetaenoic acid) and DHA (docosahexanoic acid) are the two fatty acids in this group that have been found to have potentially remarkable preventive and curative properties.

BENEFITS OF OMEGA-3 FATTY ACIDS

• Can reduce harmful cholesterol and triglycerides, and lower the risk of heart attack or stroke.
• Help reduce pain and inflammation of rheumatoid arthritis.
• Provide relief from the itching and scaling of psoriasis.
• Reduce the body's rejection of tissue grafts.
• Aid in the reduction and severity of migraine headaches.
• Fight harmful effects of prostaglandins (which lower immunity and encourage tumor growth) and help prevent breast cancer.
• Help in preventing arteriosclerosis.

BEST FISH SOURCES OF OMEGA-3

FISH	GRAMS PER 3 ½-OUNCE SERVING
Norway sardines	5.1
Chinook salmon	3.04
Atlantic mackerel	2.18
Pink salmon	1.87
Canned light albacore tuna	1.69
Sablefish	1.39
Atlantic herring	1.09
Rainbow trout (U.S.)	1.08
Pacific oyster	.84
Striped bass	.64
Channel catfish	.61
Ocean perch	.51
Cooked, canned blue crab	.46
Pacific halibut	.45
Shrimp	.39
Yellowtail flounder	.30
Haddock	.16

If you don't like fish or cannot eat it on a regular basis, fish supplements are an alternative. Ten capsules of concentrated marine lipids usually supply 1.8 g. of EPA. (A 4-ounce serving of salmon contains about 1 g.) Cod-liver oil contains EPA, too, but amounts vary according to brand, and it hasn't been shown effective in lowering blood cholesterol. Also, cod-liver oil has high amounts of vitamins A and D, which can be toxic in large amounts.

CAUTION: Potential toxicity of Omega-3 supplements is still being evaluated. Check with your doctor before starting on Omega-3 or any other supplement regimen.

98. Pasta Pitfalls

Pasta has become the "in" food of the 1980s. It is the complex carbohydrate muscle fuel that athletes load up on before competitions; the new low-fat, low-calorie dinner for dieters; the new preferred food for diabetics because it doesn't cause a rapid blood sugar rise after eating. But pastas are made from different types of flour, and different flours come from different grains, and different grains have different benefits and risks for different people (see section 114).

Perhaps the most common pasta pitfall is the most common pasta: spaghetti. Many commercial brands are not made with durum wheat, which is used to make durum flour and semolina and contains more protein than ordinary enriched pasta. Also, manufacturers tend to recommend cooking their products longer than necessary, which increases calories, depletes nutrients, and renders it more starchy and less desirable for use by diabetics. (When overcooked, pasta's sugars enter the bloodstream faster, causing insulin to overreact and bring blood sugar down, resulting in fatigue and hunger.) Pasta should be cooked *al dente*—that is, firm and slightly chewy.

Not all pasta is perfect.

Pasta packed in clear cellophane, or with large cellophane windows, is subject to nutrient loss. And any pasta containing disodium phosphate (which is added to make it quick cooking) should be avoided.

The greatest pasta pitfall is the tendency to smother it with rich, creamy sauces that are mostly fat. This can harm not only your arteries and pile on pounds, but diminish alertness. Because fat is hard to digest, blood is waylaid in the stomach for hours instead of energizing your brain.

(*Tip:* Sprinkling it with a bit of olive oil, which has been found to be a cholesterol-lowering fat, and adding some cooked clams or mussels can turn it into a really wholesome dinner.)

Eating pasta without protein can leave you feeling sluggish an hour or two later, so it's advisable to have some sort of protein for an appetizer if you are not going to add it to the pasta itself.

Keep in mind that there are two general types of pasta: one includes spaghetti, macaroni, shells, and lasagna; the other is noodles, which by law must contain at least 5½ percent egg solids. These add cholesterol and might not be advisable for individuals on a low-cholesterol diet. (Check with your doctor.) With the exception of oriental egg noodles, though, Asian noodles are *not* made with eggs. Since they look like noodles but cannot be labeled as such, they are usually marked "imitation noodles" or "alimentary paste" on packages.

If you have a gluten intolerance, you should avoid pasta made with wheat. This might sound difficult, but it isn't. Buckwheat pasta, which is gluten free, can be obtained in health food stores, as can wheatless corn pasta. There are also Chinese bean threads and cellophane noodles (made from mung beans, the cellophane noodles sometimes from seaweed); and Japanese shirataki (also made from mung beans, but with yams and other root plants that are used, too, for Japanese saifun).

CAUTION: Dried seasonings that are often sold for use with oriental noodles to make soup generally contain MSG.

99. Any Questions About Chapter 8?

I have heard that fatty fish are those most likely to contain PCBs. Is this true? And if so, wouldn't it be more dangerous to eat them?

Yes, it is true, but fatty fish also contain the largest amounts of Omega-3 fatty acids. If you enjoy eating fish, find out which ones come from unpolluted waters. The EPA (see section 145) will be able to tell you which waters are contaminated, and your local fish dealer should know where his fish came from. Generally, salmon is a safe bet.

I am a non-smoker, but because of my business I eat most of my dinners in restaurants that are filled with smoke. Are there any vitamins I can take that might help protect me from the effects of inhaling these pollutants?

Antioxidants—namely, vitamins A, C, E, and selenium—are the nutrients best capable of keeping free radicals in check. Free radicals are uncontrolled oxidations that damage cells and are formed when you inhale pollutants.

Vitamin A protects your mucous membranes (in the mouth, nose, throat, and lungs) and prevents oxidation of vitamin C, allowing it to work more effectively.

Vitamin C reduces the effects of allergy-producing substances, while fighting off potential bacterial infections. It also protects vitamins A, E, and some of the B complex from oxidation.

Vitamin E has the ability to unite with oxygen and prevent it from being converted into toxic peroxides while protecting vitamins B and C from being destroyed. It also acts as an antipollutant for the lungs.

Selenium and vitamin E must both be present to correct a potential deficiency of either.

I would suggest:

• A high-potency multiple vitamin-mineral containing 10,000 IU vitamin A and 25–50 mcg. of selenium, A.M. and P.M.
• Vitamin C, 500–1,000 mg. with zinc, 2–3 times daily.
• Vitamin E (dry form), 200–400 IU, A.M. and P.M.

These vitamins work best when taken with meals. I would also recommend that if you're eating out that often you take a calcium supplement if your multiple vitamin-mineral doesn't contain at least 100 mg. of calcium. Even calcium-rich foods are depleted of that nutrient when they are reheated, kept warm under heat lights, or subjected to other common restaurant practices.

Every time my mother tells me that I am going to get sick if I keep eating at sushi bars all the time, I wind up having to scream that she's wrong, but don't know how to prove it. Do you have any suggestions?

First of all, I would suggest you stop screaming at your mother, particularly since she is not wrong. If you are eating a steady diet of raw fish, you're depleting your body of thiamine, vitamin B_1, which is known for its beneficial effects on the nervous system and mental attitude. Your screaming might be an indication that you are low on that vitamin already.

All raw fish and shellfish contain a substance that destroys B_1, but eating a varied diet makes up for this. Sushi and sashimi are fine sources of nutrients and Omega-3 fatty acids, providing the fish is fresh and from uncontaminated waters, but I don't recommend eating them to the exclusion of other foods. If you are eating out that often, try some Italian pastas, or some Mexican rice and bean dishes for variety. They're nutritious, low in fat, can replace your lost B vitamins—and make your mother happy, too.

9

THE HAZARDS OF "HEALTH" AND HEALTHY FOODS

100. All That's Fiber Isn't Fabulous

The American Cancer Institute recommends you eat 25 to 30 g. of fiber daily; the average American eats about 15 g. Unfortunately, the average American doesn't know that:

- All fiber is not the same.
- Different fibers have different effects on the body.
- No one type should be eaten to the exclusion of the others.
- Everybody doesn't need the same type or amount of fiber in his or her diet.
- Even the best sources of fiber have nutritional hazards.
- Without a sufficient intake of liquids (6 to 8 glasses daily), fiber can be constipating.
- Large increases in fiber can be dangerous for individuals with possible nutrient deficiencies (teenagers, the elderly, anyone with an illness or existing medical problem) *and should not be made without first consulting a physician!*

101. Know Your Fiber Before You Eat It

CELLULOSE AND HEMICELLULOSES

Facts:

These absorb water and facilitate smooth functioning of the large bowel. They "bulk" waste and move it through the colon more rapidly.

Best Cellulose Sources:

Whole wheat bran, cabbage, young peas, green beans, wax beans, broccoli, brussels sprouts, cucumber skins, peppers, apples, and carrots. .

Best Hemicellulose Sources:

Whole grains, bran, cereals, mustard greens, brussels sprouts, and beet roots.

What They Can Do for You:

Help prevent constipation.

Reduce risk of appendicitis.

Offer protection against diverticulosis, spastic colon, hemorrhoids, cancer of the colon, and varicose veins.

Aid in weight loss.

Possible Hazards:

Too much in your diet can cause gas, bloating, nausea, vomiting, diarrhea, and possibly interfere with the body's ability to absorb protein, as well as such necessary minerals as zinc, calcium, iron, magnesium, and vitamin B_{12}.

CAUTION: Increased fiber may be contraindicated in certain bowel disorders. A physician should be consulted before starting any high-fiber diet.

GUMS AND PECTIN

Facts:

Primarily soluble fibers, they influence absorption in the stomach and small bowel.

They *decrease* fat absorption, and lower cholesterol levels, by binding with bile acids.

They coat the lining of the gut and delay stomach emptying.

Best Sources:

Oatmeal and other rolled oat products, dried beans, apples, citrus fruits, carrots, cauliflower, cabbage, dried peas, green beans, potatoes, squash, and strawberries.

What They Can Do for You:

Lower blood cholesterol levels.

Help reduce the risk of heart attacks and strokes.

Aid in the management of diabetes by reducing the body's need for insulin by slowing sugar absorption after a meal.

Possible Hazards:

Same as for cellulose and hemicellulose, but can also interfere with the effectiveness of certain antifungal medications containing *griseofulvin*, such as Grifulvin V, Grisactin, and Fulvicin, which are used to combat fungus infections.

LIGNIN

Facts:

Reduces the digestibility of other fibers.

Lowers cholesterol levels.

Speeds food through the gut.

Best Sources:

Bran*, breakfast cereals, eggplant, green beans, strawberries, pears, radishes, and older vegetables (as vegetables age, their lignin content rises).

What It Can Do for You:

Help reduce risk of heart disease and strokes.

Lower triglyceride levels and blood pressure.

Aid in bowel regularity.

Lower the risk of diverticulosis, hemorrhoids, and colon cancer.

Aid in weight loss by reducing the number of calories absorbed and providing a feeling of "fullness."

Possible Hazards:

Same as those for other fiber.

---

*Bran, though a good source of lignin fiber, is mostly cellulose, which *does not* have the cholesterol-lowering properties of pectin and gums.

102. Dangers in Natural Foods

Just because something is natural and edible doesn't mean it is good for you, or that it can be consumed indiscriminately. All foods are essentially chemical compounds and affect the way your body functions.

• Natural toxins are present in some of our most wholesome foods.

• Some of our most wholesome foods can destroy some of our most vital nutrients.

• Some of our most vital nutrients can interact adversely with each other and harm you!

In short, the more limited your diet, the more extensively you can jeopardize your health.

103. Healthy but Hazardous

BEEF LIVER

Beef liver is one of the richest sources of natural vitamin A, but vitamin A can be a killer if consumed in excess. Toxicity symptoms include hair loss, nausea, vomiting, diarrhea, scaly skin, blurred vision, rashes, bone pain, irregular menses, fatigue, headaches, pressure within the skull, and liver enlargement. Its excessive consumption by adults (more than half a pound daily, or 4 pounds weekly, for many months) has been linked to a painful brain disorder known as pseudotumor cerebri (PTC), and daily ingestion of as little as 4 ounces can produce toxic effects in infants. Liver is also high in cholesterol, and, because it's the detoxifying organ of the body, may contain high levels of DDT and other hazardous chemicals.

POTATOES

Potatoes are great complex carbohydrates—no-fat, nutritious suppliers of high-quality vegetable protein, vitamins (especially C), minerals, and other essential nutrients. But when potato skins turn a greenish color (because of a chlorophyll buildup), they have accumulated a dangerous chemical called solanine. Solanine, present in and around these green patches, and in eyes that have sprouted, can interfere with the transmission of nerve impulses, and cause jaundice, abdominal pain, vomiting, and diarrhea.

There is controversy about whether or not solanine is destroyed by cooking, and as long as there is doubt I wouldn't count on it. If you find that your potatoes turn green in storage or sprout eyes, remove the skin and cut away the layer of potato just under it before cooking. (Storing potatoes in paper bags and away from light, or in the refrigerator, will inhibit the buildup of solanine.)

There is also controversy between rheumatologists and nutritionists about whether or not solanine poses a particular hazard for people with arthritis and other joint diseases. Until it is resolved, I'd suggest you assume that it does and be particularly careful about the potatoes you eat if you are afflicted with any of those ailments.

NUTS AND GRAINS

These are healthy, high-protein sources of B vitamins, fiber, and energy, provided they are free of aflatoxins. Aflatoxins are the by-products of molds that grow on grains and nuts, and may be carcinogenic. (Studies have shown correlations between aflatoxin consumption from foods and increased incidences of liver cancer.)

Aflatoxin levels in susceptible foods (peanuts, for instance) are monitored by the government, but government monitoring often leaves much to be desired—namely, safety. Since cooking doesn't destroy aflatoxins, it is advisable to check nuts and grains before purchasing them (and definitely before eating them) to be sure they are not moldy, shriveled, or discolored.

MUSHROOMS

They are no-fat, low-sodium, tasty sources of niacin, potassium, and selenium, and great for dieters and cholesterol watchers, provided you don't go out and pick them in the wild. Even the most experienced wild mushroom eaters have been known to make mistakes that have caused them a variety of unpleasant symptoms (nausea, vomiting, cramps, and diarrhea), and in some cases even death. There is no foolproof way to determine the safety of a wild mushroom, and since the toxic effects of many varieties are either unknown or untreatable, it's best to buy mushrooms at your local produce market—provided they have not been treated with a bisulfite solution (see section 26).

ALFALFA SPROUTS

These sprouted seeds are terrific sources of vitamins C and K, minerals, and numerous micronutrients (often more than contained in the full-grown plant). Low in calories and high in fiber, and they are a definite plus in salads. But a little goes a long way with sprouts, particularly alfalfa ones, which can be harmful if eaten in excess.

Research has shown that overconsumption of alfalfa sprouts can cause an autoimmune form of anemia. Similar to SLE (systemic lupus erythematosus), the disease is apparently caused by a substance in the sprout that mistakenly becomes part of human protein and sets off an immunological attack against the body.

CAUTION: Anyone suffering from lupus is advised not to eat sprouts at all.

SPINACH (Swiss chard, sorrel, parsley, beet greens, rhubarb)

What could possibly be naturally hazardous about Popeye's favorite food and such deep green and leafy others? The answer is oxalic acid, a natural ingredient in these nutrient-rich vegetables and fruits (as well as chocolate) that can inhibit the absorption of their calcium and iron, and bind with calcium to make another insoluble compound that may form kidney or gallbladder stones.

Calcium-rich alternatives *without* absorption-inhibiting oxalic acid, are kale, broccoli, and collard greens, which, by the way, are also fine suppliers of B vitamins.

WHOLE-GRAIN BRAN

Even the king of fiber has a potential health hazard: phytic acid. Like oxalic acid, phytic acid can block absorption of calcium and other minerals from the grain, particularly zinc. Since recent medical findings seem to indicate that zinc may be required in the synthesis of DNA, which is the body-as-computer life chip, containing all inherited traits and directing all cell activity, anything that diminishes its intake should be considered hazardous.

If you eat a lot of whole-grain cereals with milk, you should be sure to increase your intake of zinc through other foods. (See section 128.)

104. Potentially Harmful Herbs, Teas, and Spices

Herbs and spices, generally used in small amounts as seasonings or in teas, have a disproportionately large potential for causing allergic— and even toxic—reactions in unsuspecting individuals.

All herbs and spices contain chemicals, many of which are capable of upsetting normal and essential bodily functions, especially when used in mixtures where chemicals can potentiate each other.

IMPORTANT: If you are taking any medication, I would strongly advise consulting a nutritionally oriented doctor aware of herb-drug interactions, as even small amounts of certain herbs and spices can be dangerous in combination with certain chemicals.

ACONITE

The fluid extract of the root of this plant is often mixed in warm water and drunk as tea to reduce pain, fever, inflammation of the stomach, and heart palpitations. *But in the wrong proportions it can cause heart failure.*

ALOE VERA

Though most often used as a topical ointment for healing wounds, it is frequently taken internally as a mild laxative and used in the treatment of stomach ulcers. *As an ointment it can cause hives, rashes, itching, and other allergic reactions in sensitive individuals, and it can be extremely dangerous if taken internally by pregnant women.*

BLESSED THISTLE

Used in its proper proportions in teas to break up coughs and relieve congestion, blessed thistle is known by herbalists to live up to its name. But this is not an herb for amateurs, and unless you know how to brew it properly—don't. *High doses can cause diarrhea as well as burns of the mouth and esophagus.*

CHAMOMILE

Frequently the tea of choice before bedtime, because of its sedative, stomach-settling properties, it should be drunk in moderation. *It is a highly allergenic tea, and can cause severe allergic reactions—including fatal shock—in individuals with hay fever, or those sensitive to ragweed, asters, and related plants.*

COMFREY

An herb used in teas for alleviating stomach ailments, coughs, diarrhea, arthritis, liver, and gallbladder problems. Though relatively safe, it does have a significant nutritional drawback: frequent ingestion can reduce your absorption of iron and vitamin B_{12}.

JUNIPER BERRIES

Often used as a stomach tonic, as well as a diuretic and a disinfectant of the urinary tract, juniper contains nervous system toxins. *Excessive ingestion of the berries, or beverages and tonics containing them, can cause hallucinations, among other adverse reactions.*

LEMONS

Believe it or not, the fruit that saved innumerable sailors from scurvy, and that is used for seasoning tangy teas and thirst-quenching drinks, contains citral, a substance (also present in oranges) *that can block the beneficial activity of vitamin A.*

LICORICE

Natural licorice, which comes from the root of a plant, contains glycyrrhizic acid. As an herb, it is often used as a respiratory stimulant and a laxative. As a flavoring, natural licorice is often used in candy. *Consumption of large quantities (3½ ounces) daily over long periods can cause severe hypertension and cardiac arrhythmia.* (Most American licorice candy is made with synthetic flavorings and does not pose these hazards—which is just as well, since synthetic flavorings have enough of their own.)

NUTMEG

A little sprinkled on your rice pudding won't hurt. But nutmeg, like juniper, contains nervous system toxins. *Excessive consumption can cause hallucinations, which not only won't add spice to your life, but can also endanger it.*

PENNYROYAL

This herb, often referred to as lung mint, is frequently used as a tea for curing headaches, menstrual cramps, and pain. *It can induce abortion and should therefore never be used during pregnancy.*

PEPPERMINT

An effective antispasmodic, peppermint tea has been used to treat nervousness, insomnia, cramps, and headaches. Though teas made from peppermint may be caffeine free, *they contain the same tannins that are in ordinary tea, which have been linked to high rates of cancer of the esophagus and stomach.*

ROSEMARY

Taken internally, rosemary has been shown to relieve flatulence and colic, and stimulate bile release from the gallbladder. As a spice, it is a wonderful addition to salads and sauces. But a little is all you need. *Ingestion of large quantities can be toxic.*

TARRAGON

An impressive spice that adds gourmet flavor to salads, soups, and sauces, tarragon also contains the oil estragole, *which has been shown to cause cancer in laboratory animals.*

105. Raw Foods That You Are Better Off Cooking

Cooking vegetables and fruits has been an anathema for nutritionists (myself included) and health-conscious individuals for years. But the times are changing. Increased concern about nutrition has fostered numerous studies that have revealed some startling new facts about the benefits of cooking food formerly held to be more nutritious raw.

BLUEBERRIES, BLACKBERRIES, AND RED CABBAGE

Rich in vitamin B_1 (thiamine), which is essential for keeping the nervous system, muscles, and heart functioning normally—as well as for the proper digestion of carbohydrates—blueberries, blackberries, and red cabbage are some of the many fruits and vegetables usually eaten raw, but that can be better for you if cooked. They contain enzymes that deactivate nutrients, primarily vitamin B_1, when your body tries to digest them. But heat, though ordinarily an enemy of vitamin B_1, breaks down these enzymes and allows your body to get *more* of the nutrient.

RAW PEANUTS, BEANS, AND LEGUMES

These contain enzyme inhibitors that make it difficult for your body to digest protein. Once again, heat breaks down these enzymes so you can benefit from the food's nutrients. Cooking also aids in the digestion of these foods.

106. Some Other Advantages of Cooking

You might want to think twice about ordering steak tartare or making sushi a regular part of your diet when I tell you that:

• Thorough cooking has been shown to be one of the most effective preventives against food poisoning, since it can destroy salmonella bacteria.

• Cooking lowers the fat content of all meat, fish, and poultry unless, of course, you add oil to cook them.

• Studies have shown that cooking helps remove many of the fat-soluble contaminants (PCBs, for instance) that collect in the fatty tissues of fish.

• Cooked meat is easier to digest because the molecules have already been partly broken down before reaching your stomach.

• Ground beef cooked over medium heat contains chemicals that act as *anticarcinogens* and help inactivate substances that are potential cancer-causing agents.

107. When Cooking Is Not So Hot

Though many foods might be more nutritious cooked, cooking them the wrong way can sometimes be more harmful than not eating them at all.

COOKING CONSTERNATIONS

• Foods barbecued, flame-broiled, or cooked at high temperatures are very likely to contain carcinogens.

• Cooking accelerates the oxidation of fats, producing free radical molecules that can change the metabolism and growth of body cells.

• Charcoal broiling causes the rise of smoke containing a chemical known as benzopyrene, a carcinogen, to coat the food being grilled.

CAUTION: Charcoal broiling can speed up the metabolism of certain drugs and diminish their effectiveness. Among those found most vulnerable are antiasthmatic medications containing theophylline (Elixophyllin, Marax, Quibron) and analgesics containing phenacetin, such as Darvon Compound, Emprazil, Fiorinal, Norgesic, and Soma Compound.

• Adding baking soda to cooking water can destroy the food's thiamine.
• Cooking salty, acidic, or alkaline food in aluminum pots can dissolve the metal so that it leaches into the food. This intensifies the cooking odors of cabbage, broccoli, and brussels sprouts and tends to turn potatoes yellowish.

(NOTE: The possibility of a connection between aluminum and Alzheimer's disease is still under investigation, so you would be wise to choose another type of cookware until conclusive evidence eliminates any possible link.)

• Unlined copper pots can be dangerous for cooking or storing acidic foods, or any foods cooked with wine or vinegar, as the foods can absorb this mineral, which is potentially toxic.
• Glass pots might appear hazard free, but the fact that glass lets in light can increase the loss of light-sensitive nutrients, such as vitamins B_2 (riboflavin), B_{12} (cobalamin), B_{13} (orotic acid), B_{15} (pangamic acid), C (ascorbic acid), and folic acid.
• Stainless steel pots are inadvisable if you're sensitive to certain metals that can leach into foods from pots whose inner surfaces have been damaged or scratched. Even minute amounts of nickel, for instance, can cause adverse reactions, as well as destroy vitamin C in foods.
• Thawing frozen vegetables before cooking depletes them of nutrients.

108. Cooking to Preserve Nutrients and Your Health

> Short cooking time and minimum water mean more nutrients for you!

The best way to cook foods is fast, medium, and slow. Now, hold on. This only sounds confusing.

By fast, I mean microwaving, pressure cooking, steaming, or stir-frying, which destroy fewer nutrients while thoroughly cooking foods.

By medium, I mean the temperature at which food is cooked. High temperatures (above 400° F.) tend to produce more potentially cancer-causing substances and fewer anticarcinogenic ones than medium cooking temperatures.

By slow, I mean not cooking quickly with searing heat, fast deep-frying or pan-frying, and cooking slowly over a medium flame, or roasting in a medium oven.

SOME TIPS TO KEEP IN MIND

• Vitamin C is easily destroyed by heat and oxygen, but it doesn't have to be. If you put a vegetable, for instance cabbage, in water that has been boiling actively for a minute or more, the water loses its vitamin-depleting oxygen and the cabbage retains all but about 2 percent of its vitamin C. (Putting cabbage in cold water and then bringing it to a boil depletes more than twelve times that amount of vitamin C.)

• Steaming vegetables, which means using a minimum amount of water, helps keep nutrients in and vegetables looking and tasting fresh instead of overcooked. (A small colander can turn any pot into a steamer.)

• Using non-stick pans allows you to get what you want out of foods, nutrient-wise, without having to burden your body with unnecessary cooking fats or oils. (There are even non-stick woks available for stir-frying.)

• Cooking foods, particularly poultry, soon after purchase can halt the formation of surface bacteria that spoil food rapidly, and enable you to keep the food several days longer without having to freeze it.

• Cooking meats with vegetables that contain vitamins A, C, and E (see section 128), antioxidant vitamins, slows down the chemical deterioration of the meat and keeps it tasting fresher longer.

• Saving liquids from cooked vegetables for use in soups and gravies enables you to reclaim nutrients that were lost in the water.

109. Vegetarian Vulnerabilities

There are many advantages to being a vegetarian. Among them are a diminished risk of coronary disease, heart attack, stroke, hypertension, and various forms of cancer, which has been attributed to vegetarians' low consumption of saturated animal fats and high consumption of fiber, whole grains, and vegetables. But there are disadvantages, too.

Vegetarian restrictions may cause:

- Anemia
- Impaired immunity
- Vitamin and mineral deficiencies
- An inability to metabolize necessary protein

110. The Big B_{12} Problem

Strict vegetarians, who eat no animal foods of *any* kind (no milk, cheese, eggs, dairy products) and derive their protein solely from plant sources, are very often deficient in vitamin B_{12}, which is essential for forming and regenerating red blood cells and preventing anemia.

Unfortunately, symptoms of B_{12} deficiency may not appear for five years *after the body's stores have been depleted*—which is a long time for any body to be in nutritional debt.

SUGGESTED SOLUTIONS

- A high-potency vegetarian multivitamin-mineral tablet, vitamin B_{12}, 100 mcg., and a good B complex with folic acid, taken with meals twice daily.
- Including fortified soy milk or fortified nutritional yeast in your diet. (NOTE: Brewer's yeast, baker's yeast, and live yeast are not the same as fortified nutritional yeast and do *not* supply ample amounts of vitamin B_{12}.)
- Adding seaweeds, such as dulse, kelp, and spirulina (a freshwater relative), to your meals. These are prime vegetable sources of vitamin B_{12}, as well as other nutrients, and can be prepared in a variety of ways.

CAUTION: Spirulina has a high phenylalanine content, and is contraindicated during pregnancy, and for anyone with PKU or skin cancer.

111. The Amino Acid Balancing Act

Without proper balancing of amino acids through the right combination of foods, vegetarians may suffer from a lack of *usable* protein.

In order for effective protein synthesis to occur, there must be a balance between "essential" and "nonessential" amino acids, and the essentials in proper proportion to one another. (A complete list of proper amino proportions, and answers to personal questions regarding them, can be obtained by sending a stamped self-addressed envelope to Amino Acid Research Group, P.O. Box 5277, Berkeley, CA 94705.)

For example, the essential amino acid lysine is needed for growth, tissue repair, and the production of antibodies, hormones, and enzymes. It is present in all protein-rich foods, including soy products, but is not in certain cereal proteins such as gliadin (from wheat) and zein (from corn). For vegetarians, this can present serious problems since wheat and corn are common dietary staples.

Lysine should be consumed in a 2:1 ratio to methionine (another essential amino acid). If not, a food that contains 100 percent of your lysine requirement but only 20 percent of your methionine will result in only 10 percent of the protein in that food being usable as protein by your body. (The remainder becomes fuel instead of body-tissue repair and building material.) Combining a lysine-rich food with another that's high in methionine solves the problem.

Vegetarians who find themselves troubled by an inability to concentrate, fatigue, bloodshot eyes, nausea, dizziness, hair loss, cold sores, and anemia, are usually deficient in lysine. Methionine deficiencies, characterized by the body's inability to process urine, resulting in edema (swelling due to retention of fluids in tissues) and increased susceptibility to infection, are equally common in amino acid imbalanced diets. (Cholesterol deposits, arteriosclerosis, and hair loss have also been linked to methionine deficiency.)

Because so many fruits and vegetables are either missing or low in amino acids, rendering those that are present relatively useless unless they are combined in a meal with foods high in those amino acids, the careful combining of complete and incomplete proteins (see section 91) is a vegetarian necessity.

SUGGESTED SOLUTIONS

• Vegetarian supplements. These can be obtained in liquid or powdered form and are derived from soybeans, which contain all the essential amino acids. Available without carbohydrates or fats, these supplements generally supply about 26 g. of protein an ounce (2 tablespoons), about the equivalent of a 3-ounce T-bone steak. Look for formulas modeled after naturally occurring proteins so that you can get the proper therapeutic value.

CAUTION: It is dangerous for any supplement to be used in place of food on a regular basis, taken in megadoses, or substituted for medication without the advice of a physician. Always keep supplements out of the reach of children.

112. An Apple Today Can't Keep Doctors Away

Apples are filled with fabulous pectin fiber, along with potassium, vitamin A, and other wholesome nutrients. Unfortunately, they may also be filled with daminozide, a suspected carcinogen that contains a compound (UDMH), formed by heat or digestion, that is even more potentially carcinogenic.

> Many apple products should definitely be kept out of the mouths of babes.

This chemical spray, sold under the brand name Alar, is used by numerous growers to prevent ripening apples from dropping prematurely, enhance their quality, and increase their storage life. But unlike other sprays and waxes that have been used on produce for fresh-picked sales' appeal, daminozide *cannot be washed or peeled away.* It is absorbed inside the fruit, passing on right to you its insidious residue in products made from the fruit, such as juice, sauce, cider, and in pies.

For adults who consume apple products only occasionally, the risk is considered minimal. But for infants and young children, whose bodies are growing rapidly, even a little could be hazardous.

(Most major baby food manufacturers now test all apples before use to be sure they contain no daminozide. Also, many states have passed laws prohibiting the use of daminozide in heat-processed apple products, and several manufacturers (Mott's Red Cheek, Tree Top, and Very Fine) have voluntarily refused to accept apples treated with the chemical. But with no federal prohibition of its use, there are numerous adult apple products containing daminozide being consumed by youngsters whose parents are unaware that they are feeding their children potentially carcinogenic time bombs and putting their own health in jeopardy at the same time.

Until such time as the EPA bans the use of daminozide completely, I would suggest you buy your apples only from local growers who don't use the spray, keep adult apple products out of the mouths of babes, and severely restrict your intake of juices, sauces, and other apple products that are not known to be daminozide free.

113. Crudités to Consume Cautiously

Nouvelle cuisine is fine, but certain wholesome crudités are not for everyone. Broccoli, brussels sprouts, cabbage, cauliflower, horseradish, kale, and turnips, among others, can interfere with thyroid function.

Consumption of large amounts of these cruciferous vegetables, which, ironically, have been shown to have impressive anticarcinogenic properties, can cause iodine-deficiency disease, goiter, thyroiditis, hyper- or hypofunction of the thyroid gland.

If you have an underactive thyroid gland, an excessive intake of these vegetables can worsen your condition by undermining the effectiveness of such medications as Proloid, Synthroid, and similar others. In fact, if your thyroid is underactive and you are trying to lose weight, eating large amounts of these low-calorie vegetables could be the reason you can't shake those pounds. But when these vegetables are eaten in moderation, they are great sources of nutrients and are highly recommended.

114. Half-Truths About Whole Grains

There are few finer sources of fiber, nutrients, and complex carbohydrates than whole grains. But a lot about whole grains should be taken, literally and figuratively, with a grain of salt. (In fact, cooking grains with a pinch of salt is recommended to alkalinize their acidic properties, though a side dish containing salt and thorough chewing can perform the same function.)

WHAT YOU SHOULD KNOW ABOUT GRAINS

• Bran is not a balanced food.
(It is an indigestible complex sugar that is only part of a nutrient-balanced whole grain.)

• Oats contain the highest percentage of fat of any cultivated grain.
(They also contain a natural antioxidant that retards spoilage, have been found to lower blood cholesterol levels and insulin requirements, and are a good replacement grain for individuals allergic to wheat.)

• Buckwheat groats and grits are not truly grains, and are in the same botanical family as belladonna.
(They are nonetheless fine sources of vitamin E and have been found to neutralize toxic acidic wastes in the body.)

• Corn is one of the most popular but least nutritionally complete grains.
(When popped, it has terrific fiber benefits, otherwise it should be consumed with other foods to provide any significant nutrient value.)

• Rye has the highest amount of lysine, yet contains the lowest amount of whole-grain protein.
(Its paucity of gluten is a plus for individuals allergic to that substance.)

• Millet is rich in minerals, has perhaps the most complete protein of all grains, yet is generally considered grain that's strictly for the birds.
(This underappreciated grain happens to be the only one that can be boiled like rice for main dishes, used to thicken and flavor soups and stews, made into a breakfast cereal, and remain alkaline *without* the addition of salt.)

• Long grain rice has more protein, but fewer minerals than short grain rice.
(The rices to avoid are the "instant" and "minute" varieties, which are the lowest in nutrient content.)

• All whole grain rice is called *brown* even when it is not. (Brown rice can be cream-colored, even red, but it is still the grain highest in B-complex vitamins.)
• Barley (usually available as "pearl barley") has most of its vitamins and minerals removed during milling.
(This grain makes up for its nutrient deficiencies by being extremely easy to digest and adding healthy complex carbohydrates, when mixed in soups and pilafs, to the diets of sick or elderly individuals.)

CAUTION: Excessive and exclusive consumption of whole wheat, oat, and protein-rich grains, nuts, and seeds—all of which are plentiful sources of the amino acid arginine—can be hazardous for anyone with herpes or a schizophrenic condition.

115. Finding Grains of Goodness
Buying whole grains without knowing what to look for in quality can rip you off nutritionally and economically.

A GRAIN-BUYING GUIDE

1. The grains in the bin should look whole and distinct at first glance. (Consistency of milling is a sign of quality.)
2. There should be no more than a minimum amount of unhulled or greenish, immature grains.
3. Broken or damaged grains are nutrient wipeouts, and more than a minimum number in any one bin is a good indicator of the poor quality of the lot.
4. The bin should contain no extraneous matter, such as particles of dirt or stones, and the kernels for any single grain should be all about the same size or shape.
5. Test grains at home for nutritive quality by pouring a cup of them into a pot of water. Wholesome grains will sink to the bottom. If more than 1 or 2 percent remain floating, you'd be wise to look for another supplier.

116. Getting Sour on Yogurt
In the Middle East it is known as *mast*, in Armenia *matzoon*, in Russia it is *kumyss* or *kefir*, but most of us know it as yogurt.

Originally consumed here as a health food, because of its beneficial culture *Lactobacillus bulgaricus*, which is used to ferment or curdle the milk with which it is made, yogurt has now become almost as popular as ice cream—and just about as nutritious.

Misconceptions about yogurt are as plentiful as the varieties available.

Yes, there are lots of good things to say about yogurt, but that doesn't mean all of them are true. In fact, there are a lot of "yes-buts" about yogurt that most people don't know.

YES...	BUT...
Yogurt is a good food for dieters.	It is *not* nonfattening. Plain whole-milk yogurt has virtually the same number of calories as the milk used to make it. (One cup of whole milk has 150 calories; a cup of plain whole-milk yogurt has approximately 140 calories—and some commercial brands have even more.)
Yogurt helps digestion and replaces friendly bacteria that are often destroyed during antibiotic therapies.	All brands of yogurt do not contain these beneficial bacterial cultures because many manufacturers pasteurize the yogurt *after* culturing, destroying the bacteria to extend the shelf life of their product.
Yogurt is nutritious.	It is not a complete meal any more than a glass of milk is. In fact, yogurt is slightly lower in vitamins A, C, folic acid, and magnesium than fortified milk. Unless yogurt is eaten with fresh vegetables or fruit, it's little more than a wholesome snack.

Yᴇs . . .	Bᴜᴛ . . .
Yogurt is pure and natural.	Only if it is homemade, or among a select few plain (unflavored) commercially marketed brands. Most contain stabilizers and other additives. Fruit-filled or "naturally flavored" yogurts contain added sweeteners (which are sometimes listed separately or covered under the heading "selected preserves" on labels), and often potassium sorbate, modified food starch, artificial colors and flavors as well.
Frozen yogurt has much less fat than ice cream.	It has about the same number of calories because of the added sweeteners.

117. What They Forgot to Tell You at the Health Food Store

A little bit of knowledge can be a dangerous thing when it comes to foods and supplements consumed primarily for health benefits.

For instance, we all know that vitamin A is good for the eyes. But consuming excessive amounts of liver, or downing mega A supplements daily, is more likely to produce hypervitaminosis A than to prevent or cure eye defects.

Aside from the fact that vitamins don't work alone, and that excessive or exclusive consumption of any nutrient or food can be hazardous to your health, being unaware of how even the most beneficial products from nature's pantry can backfire for you is not just asking for trouble—it is ensuring it.

ABOUT GINSENG

Ginseng is an authentic, natural, mental and physical stimulant that helps assimilate vitamins and minerals. Often called manroot because of its resemblance to the human body, it has been used around the world for centuries as a natural "upper" and an aphrodisiac. (Because of its normalizing effect on the body's metabolism, it reduces stress, which can contribute significantly to sexual performance and pleasure.) Unfortunately, many ginseng users never benefit from it. This is because they are rarely informed that vitamin C—and foods rich in vitamin C—can inhibit its effectiveness. Taking ginseng three hours before or after a vitamin C supplement, or C-rich foods, should correct this. (Also, taking a time-release vitamin C supplement makes counteraction less likely.)

ABOUT GARLIC

Garlic has been found to contain substances that reduce high blood pressure, help combat diabetes by cleaning the blood of excess glucose (which is not to suggest it be used to replace medically prescribed methods), increase immunity to bronchial infections, aid in fighting certain types of cancer, lower blood cholesterol levels, and help in the prevention of heart diseases. But it is the *oils* of these bulbs that contain the therapeutic properties. If the "odorless" pills you have been buying contain only garlic powder, you're getting a nutritional brush-off. Look for perles containing extracts of fresh garlic. They are just as odorless because they dissolve in the lower intestine, not in the stomach. But if you're concerned about your breath, taking a few natural chlorophyll tablets (which happen to have antibacterial properties that go beyond bad breath) should solve the problem.

ABOUT YEAST

Yeast is an excellent source of protein, a superior source of the natural B-complex vitamins (with the exception of B_{12}, which is bred only into fortified nutritional yeast), organic iron, trace minerals, and amino acids. But like other protein foods, yeast is high in phosphorus, which means that to reap its benefits without jeopardizing your health you should be adding extra calcium to your diet. Too much phosphorus, in case you have forgotten, can take calcium *out of the body*. And if you want your nutritional pluses from yeast to *really* rise, take a balanced B-complex supplement along with it. Together they work like a powerhouse.

ABOUT CAROB

Carob is a terrific alternative to chocolate because it is caffeine free and is much lower in fat. (Carob powder has less than .5 g. fat as opposed to cocoa powder's 3 to 5.5 g.) But by the time the manufacturers turn carob powder into carob coating for candy, they have added enough oil so that these so-called health treats have as much if not more fat per ounce than almost any commercial chocolate bar.

ABOUT SAFFLOWER OIL

Safflower oil has the highest percentage of unsaturated fats and is highest in linoleic acid (found to aid in combating cholesterol deposits and heart disease, protecting against the harmful effects of X rays, and promoting healthy skin and hair). But most buyers aren't told that it spoils easily, requires refrigeration in warm climates, and should not be used for deep-frying because its flavor is unstable under high temperatures.

ABOUT SOYBEAN OIL

Soybean oil is a strong seller—with a strong flavor—with vegetarians. The kind sold in health food stores is unrefined and highly susceptible to oxidation. Though often used in salad dressings, foods fried in it develop off-flavors quickly. (If you are going to fry food, I would recommend sesame oil. It's mild in flavor, 87 percent unsaturated, not prone to quick oxidation, and it tastes good, too.)

ABOUT POLYUNSATURATED OILS

All of them aren't the same, and though all contain high amounts of linoleic acid (necessary for producing the lecithin that lowers blood cholesterol levels), many are refined to the point that they are virtually depleted of vitamin E and other nutrients. Since the amount of vitamin E that you need is directly proportional to the amount of polyunsaturates you consume, a polyunsaturated oil with its vitamin E removed can, in effect, create a ready-made vitamin E deficiency.

118. Soy What?

Soy is the prime source of protein for vegetarians and millions of people around the world. A bean of unique taste and amazing versatility, it is used as grits and flakes for cereals and stuffings, as flour for pasta, as powder to give beverages a protein charge, as nuts for snacks, as a milk for individuals with a lactose intolerance or milk allergy, as textured vegetable protein (TVP) to form meat, chicken and fish analogs, and as curdled or fermented milk for formed bean cakes known as tofu and tempeh.

Tofu is among the most popular soy products because of its high-protein and low-fat content. (A 4-ounce piece has approximately 10 g. of protein and 5 g. of fat, only a small portion of which is saturated.) And it also contains less than 10 mg. of sodium. So, you might wonder, what could be wrong with it? Well, there are a few things.

Because of its ability to function as an all-around wholesome substitute for meat, chicken, and fish, and its lack of natural flavor, it is frequently used in recipes containing large amounts of soy sauce, which has large amounts of sodium, and fried in large amounts of oil, which imbue it with more fat than any wholesome food should have.

Soft tofu is generally preferred over hard tofu, which is unfortunate since hard tofu has the higher nutrient content. Also, tofu does not contain vitamin B_{12}, nor does it offer the dietary fiber benefits of its whole-bean parent.

Soy desserts, such as Tofutti and other soy ice creams, contain virtually no tofu. And some soy ice creams that claim to be "all natural" use refined sugar as their principal ingredient. On the other hand, these desserts are still superior to regular ice cream because of their lower percentage of saturated fat.

119. Any Questions About Chapter 9?

Are "cold pressed" oils better for you than regular ones?

No, because the words "cold pressed" on a label mean essentially nothing. Though high pressures can darken and diminish oil protein, temperatures used for the best pressed oils rarely are below 140° F. In fact, many allegedly cold pressed oils are actually chemically extracted, deodorized, and bleached. Because these words have been used so frequently by disreputable manufacturers, many reputable ones won't even put the term on their labels.

High-quality oils are unrefined; just pressed, filtered, and then bottled. They might appear slightly cloudy, but retain the color, smell, and flavor of the seed, bean, or nut they came from. They're the ones you want.

My husband and I are vegetarians, and occasionally make meatless burgers from mixes that I get at the health food store. They don't seem to bother him, but I seem to break out in hives, or get flushed and itchy, mostly on nights that we eat them. Do natural meat analogs contain substances that can cause allergic reactions?

They do indeed, especially if you are allergic to any grains, such as wheat, oats, barley, millet, or legumes (soybeans, peas, lentils), or nuts, which are often used in varying combinations in meat analogs. Check ingredients carefully, because many also add egg to their formulas along with different dehydrated vegetables. In fact, some imply they are totally natural (may even be labeled as such) and are sold in health food stores even though they contain carrageenan, MSG, artificial flavors, and other additives—any of which might be causing your after-dinner discomforts.

Is there any way to tell if the yogurt I'm eating really has the live cultures I want for replacing the good bacteria in my system?

Yes, there is, and it's almost as easily done as said. Mix a few tablespoons of your plain yogurt with a cup of warmed (not boiled) milk. Leave the mixture overnight in a warm place (over the pilot light on the range will do). If your yogurt passes the test and has live cultures, the milk will have thickened somewhat by morning. If your yogurt fails, the milk will just be...milk. If so, change your brand.

I have been told by my doctor that soybeans are difficult to digest. I find this difficult to believe. I think he just says things like this because he doesn't approve of vegetarianism.

You might be better off finding yourself a nutritionally oriented physician (see section 143), but your present doctor does know his beans. Whole soybeans are very difficult to digest, basically because of their high protein and oil content. They can also be extremely gaseous. Tofu, on the other hand, which is made from soybeans, is very easy to digest, nongaseous, and can provide you with virtually all nutrients of the whole bean.

I've heard that frozen vegetables have more vitamins than fresh ones. Could this possibly be true?

In many cases it is. Vegetables begin to lose vitamins, particularly vitamin C, as soon as they're picked. By freezing or even canning them immediately, they tend to retain more vitamins than if they are exposed to lengthy storage and shipping time (yes, in spite of losses incurred by processing). Frozen vegetables, though, retain more vitamins than those that are canned, because vitamins, especially water-soluble ones, are more nutritionally stable in cold than in heat.

I use walnuts quite often in salads and breads, so to save time I buy them already shelled. Are they any less nutritious this way?

They are not only less nutritious, they are more potentially hazardous to your health. Because of their high oil content, the removal of their shells leaves them vulnerable to rancidity. And depending upon how they are processed, you are left vulnerable to the fumigants that are used in their processing.

Ethylene gas, whose fumes are irritating to membranes and whose ingestion as a solvent can cause liver and kidney damage, is generally used to loosen the walnuts from their shells. After shelling, the nuts are protected from spoilage (though you're not) by methyl bromide, which is a potential central nervous system depressant, and then blanched by a dip in hot dye or glycerine and sodium carbonate, which in excessive amounts has been shown to increase acidity and cause serious kidney damage in dogs. Since color is considered important to sales, walnuts are also often bleached with chloride of lime and sodium carbonate.

If you're buying shelled nuts, I would suggest you steer clear of those that have been overly processed. Natural food stores are your best bet for purchasing these. Look for solid kernels. If they feel soft or rubbery, the nuts are probably old and possibly rancid. Avoid any kernels whose insides are beginning to turn gray. This is an indication that oils are coming out and rancidity has begun.

What's the difference between parboiled, polished, and converted white rice?

Polished white rice, the sort you get in most Chinese restaurants, is rice that has been depleted of a large portion of its nutrients, particularly B vitamins, through a process that is used to make its protein more digestible. (This is a dubious trade-off for Westerners, whose diets are generally oversupplied with protein.)

Parboiled and converted white rice, on the other hand, is processed so that nutrients in the bran (outer layer) are essentially pushed into the endosperm, thereby retaining many more of the grain's natural vitamins and minerals.

What precisely is the big difference between soluble and insoluble fiber?

To be as precise as possible, soluble fiber interferes with the absorption of fats and slows down the absorption of carbohydrates into the body. (Examples: oat bran, legumes, citrus fruits.) Insoluble fiber is a tougher variety. It doesn't break down in water, but it does absorb it, causing waste to move through and out at a quicker pace. (Examples: wheat bran, whole grains, beans.)

The important point to remember is that the more refined a food is, the less fiber it has. In other words, applesauce would have half as much fiber as a raw apple, and white bread has about eight times less than whole wheat.

I'd like to increase the fiber in my diet, but I hate eating salads. Could you give me some suggestions on what foods supply the most in minimum amounts?

Sufficient fiber can be obtained by eating small amounts of a variety of foods. If you eat 2 slices of whole wheat bread, 2 pieces of fruit (one citrus), a cup of legumes, a cup of vegetables, and half a cup of high fiber cereal daily, you'd be getting all you need.

But if you are not prepared to make significant dietary changes yet, and following any sort of regimen on a daily basis is not for you, the following foods will give you the most in minimum portions:

- One cup of baked beans = approximately 18.5 g.
- Two dried figs = approximately 18.5 g.
- One cup of green peas = approximately 11 g.
- Half a cup of bran cereal = approximately 10 g.
- Half a cup of peanuts, or one banana = approximately 6 g.

What's the difference between "extra virgin," "virgin," and "pure" olive oil?

The cholesterol-lowering benefits of olive oil come from the fact that it is the most easily absorbed monounsaturated fat around. _Extra virgin oil_ is the best quality, made from the choicest olives, and by law may not contain more than 1 percent of unsaturated fatty acid. _Virgin oil_ may contain up to 3.3 percent unsaturated acid. _Pure olive oil_ is usually a blend of virgin or extra virgin oils and may contain some impurities, though not of any real consequence.

Extra virgin and virgin are more costly than pure olive oil, but a little goes a long way and provides a high health return. You can use extra virgin or virgin olive oil, with a little lemon, as a fine replacement for butter sauces by drizzling a small amount over cooked vegetables, or adding some garlic to it and spreading it on crunchy Italian bread.

I have just recently heard of a grain called triticale. Do you know anything about it?

Enough to recommend its use. It is a man-made hybrid grain, a cross between wheat and rye, and with more nutritive value than both. In fact, its biological value has been found to be better than that of soybeans. As a whole grain it's generally cooked as pilaf or added to soups; as a flour it's used for bread, cakes, muffins, etc. It is low in gluten, but not low enough to recommend it for anyone with an allergy to gluten. Triticale products are difficult to find in many areas, but you can write to the main commercial supplier, Arrowhead Mills (Box 866, Hereford, TX 79045), for the name of a local distributor.

10

CAUTIONS
À LA CARTE

120. Food Poisoning Is Alive and Well

> Over 8,000 Americans die from foodborne infections every year!

Foods deteriorate because of microbiologic, physical, chemical, or enzyme-induced decay. Food processing, for better or worse, can eliminate or reduce natural and added toxins, destroy harmful parasites, and maintain nutrient quality and flavor. Nonetheless, food poisoning is still alive and well and killing people every year—mostly because of human error.

COMMON TYPES OF FOOD POISONING

Botulism

This type of food poisoning is caused by eating food that contains poison or toxin produced by bacteria growing *in the food*. Though rare (about 10 to 15 cases annually in the United States) botulism can be, and frequently is, deadly. Most cases are the result of improperly home-canned foods, although a few have been traced to commercially processed foods.

Symptoms: Mild stomach upset and general malaise usually appear some 18 to 48 hours after eating the poisoned food. These are followed quickly by dizziness and headache, with blurred or double vision; general muscular weakness, difficulty in swallowing and speaking; respiratory failure and coma. Death is caused by respiratory paralysis. (The odds of survival depend on the amount of poison ingested in relation to the person's body weight and how quickly emergency treatment can be given.)

If botulism is suspected, the victim should be given absolutely nothing by mouth and rushed to the hospital. Antitoxin is not always available at hospitals, but can be obtained by having your doctor phone the 24-hour botulism hot line at the Center for Disease Control in Atlanta for information on the nearest supply. The line is for use *only by physicians* who have diagnosed the case.

Prevention tips:

• Never eat or even taste food from a swollen can or jar.
• If the contents of any can or jar are foamy, moldy, or have a bad odor, dispose of them *immediately.* (Be sure there's no chance they will even be *tasted* by pets.)
• Never taste home-canned vegetables before cooking them. (Letting them boil for a few minutes will destroy any botulism bacteria.)
• If you are unsure of how to go about home canning, contact your local Agricultural Extension Service for reliable information— or else can the idea completely.

Staphylococcal Food Poisoning

More common, but less dangerous than botulism, this type is also caused by eating food containing poison or toxin produced by bacteria growing *in the food*. (NOTE: For infants, elderly people, and anyone suffering from other illnesses, this type of food poisoning *can* be fatal.) The staphylococcus bacteria is harmful only when it is allowed to contaminate and multiply in food that has been improperly stored, cooked, or handled.

Symptoms: Nausea, general malaise, vomiting and/or diarrhea usually appear anywhere from 1 to 6 hours after eating a food contaminated with staphylococcus. Vomiting need not be induced, but should not be inhibited, mainly because vomiting and diarrhea can rid your body of the toxin within a day or two. When initial symptoms subside, you can drink warm mild fluids (broth, tea, etc.), and then stay on a bland diet for a few days. Special medications are generally not recommended, but you should check with your physician to be sure.

Prevention tips:

• Don't eat raw meat.
• Keep raw foods refrigerated. (If poultry or meat is contaminated with staphylococcus, the bacteria will multiply rapidly at room temperature—and the staphylococcus toxin is *not* destroyed by heating.
• Thaw meat and poultry in the refrigerator, microwave, or in a plastic wrap under cold water, quickly.

Salmonellosis

This type of food poisoning is an infection caused by eating food containing organisms that multiply *in the body*. It is often caused by undercooked poultry, insufficiently reheated leftovers, raw or rare meat, contaminated eggs and other dairy products, putting warm stuffing into a raw turkey and allowing it to remain uncooked (even though refrigerated) overnight. (The cold cannot penetrate the center of the turkey fast enough to kill rapidly multiplying salmonella.) Frequently misdiagnosed as an intestinal virus, the diarrheal infection caused by this bacteria may leave a legacy of serious chronic ailments, such as arthritis, kidney damage, heart problems, and intestinal damage that interferes with the ability to absorb nutrients, leaving victims with impaired immunity to numerous other illnesses.

Symptoms: Abdominal cramps, watery diarrhea, chills, and possibly fever can appear anywhere from 6 hours to a couple of days after eating the contaminated food because it takes time for the bacteria to grow in your intestinal tract. A physician should be called, since the infection could be dangerous and lead to complications. Antibiotics may or may not be required, depending upon your doctor's assessment of the condition. (Frighteningly, new research indicates that many strains of salmonella bacteria have become antibiotic-resistant, making the infection more dangerous today than in the past.) Diagnosis is generally confirmed by a stool sample.

Prevention tips:

• Scrub all surfaces on which you cut raw poultry before putting any other food there.
• Before handling other food, wash your hands and utensils after cutting raw poultry or meat.
• Cook all poultry thoroughly. (The center must reach 165° F. to kill salmonella bacteria.)
• Keep foods either hot (above 165° F.) or cold (below 40° F.), and don't let them stand at in-between temperatures, particularly warm ones, for more than 2 hours.
• Don't let hot foods cool on the counter. Gradual cooling allows prime time for salmonella growth. Food should be cooled to 40° F. within 4 hours. (If you've made a large pot of stew or chili that won't cool fast enough, divide it into smaller containers.)
• Never leave meat or poultry to defrost on the counter.
• Don't use eggs that have cracks in them.

Seafood Poisoning

There are two types of seafood poisoning: mytilotoxism, which comes from eating mollusks such as mussels, clams, and oysters that have fed on certain toxic microorganisms; and ciguatera poisoning, which can be caused by eating any contaminated seafood. Both types are serious and potentially fatal.

Symptoms: For mytilotoxism, symptoms appear very quickly, usually within half an hour. Nausea and vomiting is followed by paralysis that begins in the outer extremities and spreads to the rest of the body. Emergency treatment is required. If vomiting hasn't occurred, it should be induced, and the victim taken to the hospital. If you or others have eaten the shellfish, induce vomiting and proceed immediately to the hospital—even if no symptoms are apparent.

Symptoms of ciguatera poisoning usually take 3 to 5 hours to appear. They include nausea, fatigue, giddiness, and increased salivation and sweating. Headache, dizziness, and difficulty in breathing follow. Respiratory failure can occur if the victim is not given emergency treatment. CPR or other respiratory resuscitation may be required en route to the hospital.

Prevention tip:

• Don't eat your own catch if you don't know what your own catch has been eating. (Commercial fisheries have much better surveillance and knowledge of what they bring in from the sea, but be forewarned that current law still does not require inspection of fish and shellfish or of the plants in which they are processed. I'm not implying that you should avoid fish, just suggesting that you would be wise to buy only from reputable suppliers who know where their fish are coming from.)

121. Protecting Yourself at Home and in Restaurants

Eliminating all the bacteria that cause food poisonings is impossible, but stopping their growth, killing them at the proper time, and preventing them from doing their dirty work are not.

PRECAUTIONS FOR ALL OCCASIONS

• Never taste meat, poultry, or fish while it is cooking. (All it takes is a spoonful of uncooked bouillabaisse to let an unwanted parasite slip through your lips or put a germ of your own in the pot.)
• Avoid using the same spoon more than once for tasting food while preparing, cooking, or serving.
• Never eat or serve food directly from a jar or can; saliva may contaminate the remaining food. (This can be particularly hazardous for infants.)
• Always keep uncooked and cooked foods containing eggs in the refrigerator.
• Don't hold food for more than 2 to 3 hours in an automatic oven before cooking.
• Cutting boards, meat grinders, blenders, and can openers should be washed thoroughly after each use. (Chlorine laundry bleach in the proportion recommended on the package is an effective destroyer of bacteria.)

• Never partially cook meat or poultry one day and complete cooking the next.

• Always wash your hands before cooking and eating. (The worst organisms for foodborne illnesses are fecally transmitted.)

• Be wary of eating food that has been prepared by someone smoking. (Smoking hazards aside, saliva might have gotten on her fingers, from the cigarette between her lips, and it can transmit unwanted bacteria to you.)

• Avoid restaurants where soups are served warm instead of hot, and salads tepid instead of chilled. (The longer food sits in temperatures conducive to bacterial growth, the more likely the presence of harmful bacteria.)

122. Is That Still Okay to Eat?

How many times have you opened your refrigerator, freezer, or pantry and wondered whether or not something was still okay to eat and wound up convincing yourself that it was?

How many times have you told yourself, "When in doubt throw it out" and have?

Foods don't have to be toxic to be dangerous.

If you have done more of the eating than the throwing out, you're playing a risky nutritional game. Foods don't have to be toxic to sabotage your body. They can quite efficiently undermine you physically and emotionally simply by depriving you of nutrients, or by sneakily plying you with relatively harmless bacteria that slowly but surely can weaken your immune system, leaving you vulnerable to innumerable, avoidable ailments.

Keeping yourself out of nutritional danger is knowing what and when foods could be harmful—and not eating them.

123. Learn the Dating Game

Most processed foods are dated in a code that only the manufacturer can decipher. Some perishable foods, however, are required by law to have what is known as an "open date" that consumers can understand. Unfortunately, there are four kinds of open dates (blind dates would be a more appropriate description), and it's a rare consumer who understands any of them. But learning how can make a big difference to your health.

TRANSLATIONS FOR CONSUMERS

• Dairy products, cold cuts, fresh fruit juices, and bakery goods usually have a "sell by" date, indicating that the product should not be sold after that date (though bakery goods often are, at reduced prices).

Translation: Unless the product can be frozen, you shouldn't keep it for more than 2 to 3 days.

• Canned and frozen foods have a "packed on" date, which isn't too helpful unless you know how long the food will remain fresh, which most of us don't.

Translation: Use the frozen foods within 3 to 4 months of the date, canned foods within a year. There is no health danger in keeping them longer, but there is no nutritional point to it either.

• Products marked "best if used by" mean that the manufacturer backs their quality and freshness up to that date.

Translation: It is not dangerous to use the product after the date—unless, of course, it turns moldy (see section 124)—but don't count on getting the same nutrition from it.

• Any foods that have an "expiration (EXP)" date should be taken seriously. If the manufacturer doesn't want you to eat it, that's a good enough reason not to.

Translation: If you've passed the date, dump the product.

124. Mind Those Molds

The refrigerator is a great spawning ground for molds because they can tolerate low temperatures. But these greenish-grayish intruders are not budding penicillin sources; they are powerful troublemakers that can accelerate food spoilage and produce poisons.

MUST-KNOWS ABOUT MOLD

• Never sniff moldy food. (Molds can cause allergic reactions and produce respiratory problems.)

• Foods heavily covered with mold should be carefully wrapped in a paper towel (you don't want any seditious spores let loose in your refrigerator) and discarded immediately. The area where the moldy food was should be cleaned thoroughly and all nearby foods carefully examined.

• A small moldy spot on cheese, hard salami, or smoked turkey can be cut off and the food saved, provided you cut off *at least an inch around and below the mold spot*, and rewrap the food in fresh paper. (Moldy bacon, hot dogs, sliced luncheon meats, meat pies, canned hams, and baked chicken should be thrown out.)

• Spots of surface mold on firm vegetables, such as carrots and cabbage, can be cut away and the vegetables will still be safe to eat raw or cooked. Soft vegetables (tomatoes, cucumbers, lettuce, etc.) should be discarded if they show signs of mold growth.

• Discard any moldy soft cheese, cottage cheese, cream, sour cream, yogurt, and individual cheese slices.

• Moldy bread as well as other baked goods should be discarded. (If one slice of bread has begun to green, you can be sure the mold is working its way through the loaf.)

• Dried nuts, beans, rice, whole grains, flour, corn, and peanut butter should be tossed out if there are signs of mold, as they can be extremely hazardous to your health.

125. How Long Will It Keep?

• Raisins in an airtight container, in a cool place, will keep in prime condition for more than 6 months.

• Grapes will stay fresh in the refrigerator for 3 to 5 days.

• Herbs and spices have volatile oils that oxidize easily. If stored in small jars, tightly covered, and kept away from heat, humidity, and light, they'll keep nicely for at least a year.

• Whole wheat flour will usually go rancid within 1 to 2 months unless stored in the refrigerator or frozen.

• A peanut butter sandwich will keep for 2 days without refrigeration.

• Cooked wild rice will keep for only a week in the refrigerator, but will last several months if frozen.

• Beer in cans will begin to deteriorate in 3 months; in bottles, 5 months.

• Nuts will keep for a year or longer if frozen in tight containers.

• Cooked beans, tightly covered, will keep for up to 5 days in the refrigerator.

• Eggplant will keep fresh for about a week.

• Green onions and chives should be refrigerated and used within a few days after purchase.

• Soft unripened cheeses, such as cottage, cream, or Neufchâtel, should be refrigerated and used within a few days after purchase or "sell by" date.

• Ripened and cured cheese will keep in the refrigerator for several weeks if protected from mold contamination.

• Though many cheeses are damaged by freezing, certain varieties can be frozen for 6 months if they are cut into small pieces (not over an inch thick) or grated, and wrapped in moistureproof freezer paper or stored in airtight containers. (Cheeses that are among those most suitable for freezing in small pieces are brick, Camembert, Cheddar, Edam, Gouda, mozzarella, Muenster, Port du Salut, provolone, and Swiss.

• Fresh-chilled or packaged poultry should be used within 1 to 2 days of purchase.

• Refrigerated egg yolks or whites, stored tightly covered, should still be used within 1 to 2 days.

• Fresh prepackaged meat should be stored, unopened, in the refrigerator in the original wrapping no longer than 2 days. (Larger cuts, such as roasts, may stay 3 to 4 days.) Without rewrapping, meat will stay fresh in the freezer for 1 to 2 weeks. (For longer storage, the package must be overwrapped with special freezer paper or foil.)

• Frozen meat should be stored at 0° F. or lower immediately after purchase to prevent loss of quality and bacterial growth.

• Fresh meat should be used within 2 to 4 days of purchase for optimum quality.

• Ground meats should be used within 1 to 2 days.

• Fresh beef should be kept frozen no longer than a year.

• Fresh veal and lamb should be kept frozen no longer than 9 months.

• Fresh pork should be kept frozen no longer than 6 months.

• Ground beef, veal, and lamb should be kept frozen no longer than 4 months.

• Ground pork should be kept frozen no longer than 3 months.

• Fresh pork sausage should be used within 1 week or kept frozen no longer than 60 days. (Smoked sausage should be used within 3 to 7 days.)

• Bacon and frankfurters will keep 5 to 7 days in the refrigerator; 1 month in the freezer.

• A whole smoked ham will keep 1 week in the refrigerator; 2 months in the freezer.

• Ham slices will keep 3 to 4 days in the refrigerator; 2 months in the freezer.

• Corned beef will keep 1 week in the refrigerator; 2 weeks in the freezer.

• Leftover cooked meat will keep 4 to 5 days in the refrigerator; 2 to 3 months in the freezer.

126. Portions of Cautions

No matter how nutritious a food is and how important individual nutrients are, there will always be times, situations, and metabolic conditions where cautions and special adjustments are advised. I suggest that you read the following list carefully for your own well-being. It can help you reap benefits and sidestep risks that may often be just opposite sides of the same nutritional coin.

• Whole wheat flour contains difficult-to-digest carbohydrates that are attacked by bacteria in the large intestine, frequently causing gas and diarrhea.

• Many salt substitutes contain potassium chloride, which can be hazardous in large amounts and should not be used without first consulting your physician or a nutritionally oriented doctor (see section 143).

• Overconsumption of vitamin B_1 (thiamine) can affect thyroid and insulin production, and might cause loss of other B vitamins. (See section 128 for natural sources of thiamine.)

• An insufficiency of vitamin A in your diet can lead to loss of vitamin C and a weakened immune system.

• Don't eat raw eggplant; it could contain toxic solanine. (Cooking destroys solanine.)

• Ingestion of large amounts of vitamin B_2 (riboflavin) without sufficient amounts of vitamins A, C, E, and selenium in your diet, may cause a sensitivity to sunlight.

• Don't eat raw egg whites. They deactivate the body's biotin.

• Large doses of vitamin C wash out B_{12} and folic acid, so be careful about taking C supplements—particularly if you are a vegetarian—without the compensation of sufficient B_{12} and folic acid to meet your minimum requirement.

• If you have a medical history of convulsive disorders or hormone-related cancer, high intakes of folic acid for extended periods of time are not recommended.

• Excessive consumption of foods rich in PABA (para-aminobenzoic acid) can have a negative effect on the liver, kidneys, and heart in certain individuals.

• Anyone with sickle-cell anemia, hemochromatosis, or thalasseemia should not take iron supplements, eat large amounts of iron-rich foods, or cook his meals in cast-iron pots.

• Large amounts of caffeine from coffee, colas, or chocolate can inhibit iron absorption and also create an inositol shortage in the body.

• Anyone with kidney malfunction should not eat large quantities of magnesium-rich foods. Over 3,000 mg. daily can be dangerous. (Keep in mind that just 2 cups of roasted almonds supply more than 700 mg.)

• Milk is not a good source of iron, which is necessary for the metabolization of B vitamins.

• It is possible that large amounts of vitamin C might reverse the anticoagulant activity of the blood thinner warfarin, commonly prescribed as the drug Coumadin.

• Anyone taking thyroid medication should be aware that kelp also affects that gland. If you have been using both, a consultation with your doctor is advisable. You might need *less* prescription medicine than you think.

• If you take cortisone or aldosterone drugs (Aldactone, Prednisone, etc.) you *lose* potassium and *retain* sodium. Check with your doctor for proper diet restructuring and supplements.

• If you're trying to increase the zinc in your diet, be sure you are getting enough vitamin A for it to be effective.

• Foods high in folic acid and PABA might inhibit the effectiveness of sulfonamides such as Gantrisin.

• Large amounts of raw cabbage can cause an iodine deficiency and throw off thyroid production in individuals with existing low-iodine intakes.

• Milk that contains synthetic vitamin D can deplete the body of magnesium.

• The artificial sweetener aspartame (NutraSweet) contains phenylalanine, which may raise blood pressure, and should *not* be used by anyone taking MAO inhibitors.

• If you eat a lot of protein, be sure your diet includes a substantial amount of B-complex vitamins. (Surprisingly, even B_{12}, which is ample in high-protein foods, is also necessary because it works synergistically with the other B vitamins.)

• If you drink alcohol regularly, be sure that you're getting substantial amounts of vitamin B_{12} in your diet.

• If you eat out a lot, you need to add more calcium to your diet.

• If you have an ulcer, keep away from papaya and raw pineapple, and don't use papain as a food tenderizer.

• Excessive zinc intake can result in iron and copper losses.

• Anyone suffering from Wilson's disease is susceptible to copper toxicity.

• Don't boil fluoridated water more than 10 minutes. (Boiling drives off chlorine and other contaminates, but it concentrates the fluorides to an unhealthy degree.)

• Eating large mouthfuls of food can be particularly hazardous if you're taking tranquilizers such as Compazine and Thorazine, since these drugs tend to reduce the ability to cough.

• Don't eat foods that are high in purines if you are prone to gout attacks. (Purines are found mainly in fatty meats and poultry, scallops, anchovies, clams, organ meats, and vegetables such as spinach, lentils, mushrooms, peas, and asparagus, as well as in condiments, rich pastries, fried foods, and alcohol.)

• Some antihypertensive medications can cause a buildup of potassium, while others (particularly thiazide diuretics) deplete it. Be sure you know which your drug is doing and consult your doctor about adjusting your diet and supplements accordingly.

• The gluten in wheat, rye, and barley may aggravate arthritic conditions in certain individuals, and is contraindicated for anyone with celiac disease.

• Calcium can interfere with the effectiveness of tetracycline.

• Too much manganese can reduce the utilization of your body's iron.

• If you go off the Pill in order to become pregnant, do NOT eat large amounts of vitamin A–rich foods (see section 128) or take vitamin A supplements, but do increase the folic acid in your diet. (Too much vitamin A and too little folic acid have, under these circumstances, been associated with birth defects.)

• Iodine can worsen a dermatological condition, so avoid highly salted foods (see section 93) and any that use iodized salt.

• Heavy milk drinkers and meat eaters need to increase the manganese in their diets.

• High-protein, low-carbohydrate diets can diminish your production of two essential hormones: thyroid and norepinephrine.

• Sudden stopping of a high-protein, low-carbohydrate diet can cause a rapid drop in potassium and magnesium, and result in heart rhythm irregularity.

• Chocolate can cause anal itching.

• Avoid mixed baby food dinners that might contain modified starch. Many young infants cannot digest starches. Undigested starches can cause diarrhea, which can keep an infant from absorbing necessary nutrients.

• Tomatoes should not be left to ripen in the sun. They'll lose most of their vitamin C and other nutrients.

• Bulgar wheat is not a whole wheat product unless the granules still have their dark brown bran coating.

• Potatoes should not be washed before storage nor refrigerated; storing them at temperatures below 40 to 50° F. can convert some of the starch to sugar.

• Sweets eaten between meals can be more damaging to teeth than those eaten with meals.

• Honey can cause botulism in infants because of their undeveloped digestive systems.

• Anticoagulant (blood-thinning) medications can be dangerously undermined by daily consumption of such vitamin K–rich foods as cabbage, lettuce, asparagus, turnip greens, and spinach.

• Comfrey tea, used frequently to soothe stomachs and alleviate ulcer pain, contains cancer-causing alkaloids.

• Taking antibiotics too soon after—or not long enough before— meals, can prevent them from reaching adequate levels of effectiveness to cure the disease or infection for which they have been prescribed.

• Pasta packaged in containers with a clear viewing window can lose up to half of its riboflavin in 24 hours at room temperature.

• Heavy consumption of soybeans can reduce the effectiveness of thyroid medications.

• A diet *too* high in fiber-rich foods can interfere with your body's ability to use calcium, magnesium, iron, and zinc.

127. International Cuisine Cautions

Many foreign foods have been found to offer amazing health benefits. For example:

• Japanese miso soup, made from fermented soybeans and grains, seems to reduce stomach cancer.

• Indian yogurt is a natural antibiotic that has been helpful in lowering cholesterol levels and in the treatment of hepatitis, gallstones, and kidney disorders.

• Italian olive oil is highly *monounsaturated* and has been shown to surpass all polyunsaturated oils in helping to prevent heart disease.

• Mexican corn and beans provide low-fat, high-fiber protein with large amounts of calcium (the corn is steeped in limewater) and other nutrients, and chili peppers have been found helpful in fighting asthma, bronchitis, and sinusitis. (The American Heart Association recommends salsa as a low-salt condiment.)

• Chinese mushrooms, particularly shiitake and enoki mushrooms, appear to contain powerful stimulators of the immune system.

But even the best international cuisines have their nutritional drawbacks. And when you are eating out, they should definitely be kept in mind.

INDIAN FOOD: Steer clear of dishes that are drenched in ghee.

JAPANESE FOOD: Watch out for smoked foods, which are high in nitrates, and dishes cooked with large amounts of high-sodium soy sauce.

ITALIAN FOOD: Beware of deleterious pasta smothered in rich cheese, cream, and butter sauces.

MEXICAN FOOD: Keep away from commercially prepared refried beans that are usually made with lard.

CHINESE FOOD: Soups can be hazardous since they're almost always prepared beforehand and laden with MSG. Also, adding extra soy sauce to any dish is dangerous since most are already prepared with this high-sodium condiment.

128. Do You Know the Foods That Supply Your Nutrients?

A QUICK VITAMIN, MINERAL, AND AMINO ACID REFERENCE LIST

VITAMIN	BEST NATURAL SOURCES
Vitamin A	Fish-liver oil, liver, carrots, green and yellow vegetables, eggs, milk and dairy products, margarine, yellow fruits
Vitamin B_1 (thiamine)	Dried yeast, rice husks, whole wheat, oatmeal, peanuts, pork, most vegetables, bran, milk
Vitamin B_2 (riboflavin)	Milk, liver, kidney, yeast, cheese, leafy green vegetables, fish, eggs
Vitamin B_6 (pyridoxine)	Brewer's yeast, wheat bran, wheat germ, liver, kidney, heart, cantaloupe, cabbage, blackstrap molasses, milk, eggs, beef
Vitamin B_{12} (cobalamin)	Liver, beef, pork, eggs, milk, cheese, kidney

VITAMIN	BEST NATURAL SOURCES
Vitamin B_{12} (orotic acid)	Root vegetables, whey, the liquid portion of soured or curdled milk
Vitamin B_{15} (pangamic acid)	Brewer's yeast, whole brown rice, whole grains, pumpkin seeds, sesame seeds
Vitamin B_{17} (laetrile)	A small amount of laetrile is found in the whole kernels of apricots, apples, cherries, peaches, plums, and nectarines
Biotin (coenzyme R or vitamin H)	Nuts, fruits, brewer's yeast, beef liver, milk, kidney, unpolished rice
Vitamin C (ascorbic acid)	Citrus fruits, berries, green and leafy vegetables, tomatoes, cauliflower, potatoes, sweet potatoes
Calcium pantothenate (pantothenic acid, pantothenol, vitamin B_5)	Meat, whole grains, wheat germ bran, kidney, liver, heart, green leafy vegetables, brewer's yeast, nuts, chicken, crude molasses
Choline	Egg yolk, brain, heart, green leafy vegetables, yeast, liver, wheat germ (and, in small amounts, in lecithin)
Vitamin D (calciferol, viosterol, ergosterol)	Fish-liver oils, sardines, herring, salmon, tuna, milk and dairy products
Vitamin E (tocopherol)	Wheat germ, soybeans, vegetable oils, broccoli, brussels sprouts, leafy greens, spinach, enriched flour, whole wheat, whole-grain cereals, eggs
Vitamin F (unsaturated fatty acids: linoleic, linolenic, and arachidonic)	Vegetable oils (wheat germ, linseed, sunflower, safflower, soybean, and peanut), peanuts, sunflower seeds, walnuts, pecans, almonds, avocados

VITAMIN	BEST NATURAL SOURCES
Folic acid (folacin)	Deep green leafy vegetables, carrots, tortula yeast, liver, egg yolk, cantaloupe, apricots, pumpkins, avocados, beans, whole wheat and dark rye flour
Inositol	Liver, brewer's yeast, dried lima beans, beef brains and heart, cantaloupe, grapefruit, raisins, wheat germ, unrefined molasses, peanuts, cabbage
Vitamin K (menadione)	Yogurt, alfalfa, egg yolk, safflower oil, soybean oil, fish-liver oils, kelp, leafy green vegetables
Niacin (nicotinic acid, niacinamide, nicotinamide)	Liver, lean meat, whole wheat products, brewer's yeast, kidney, wheat germ, fish, eggs, roasted peanuts, the white meat of poultry, avocados, dates, figs, prunes
Vitamin P (C complex, citrus bioflavonoids, rutin, hesperidin)	The white skin and segment part of citrus fruit (lemons, oranges, grapefruit); also in apricots, buckwheat, blackberries, cherries, and rose hips
PABA (para-amino-benzoic acid)	Liver, brewer's yeast, kidney, whole grains, rice, bran, wheat germ, molasses

MINERAL	BEST NATURAL SOURCES
Calcium	Milk and milk products, all cheeses, soybeans, sardines, salmon, peanuts, sunflower seeds, dried beans, green vegetables
Chlorine	Table salt, kelp, olives

MINERAL	BEST NATURAL SOURCES
Chromium	Meat, shellfish, chicken, corn oil, clams, brewer's yeast
Cobalt	Milk, kidney, liver, meat, oysters, clams
Copper	Dried beans, peas, whole wheat, prunes, calf and beef liver, shrimp and most other seafood
Fluorine	Seafood and gelatin
Iodine (iodide)	Kelp, vegetables grown in iodine-rich soil, onions, all seafood
Iron	Pork liver, beef kidney, heart and liver, farina, raw clams, dried peaches, red meat, egg yolk, oysters, nuts, beans, asparagus, molasses, oatmeal
Magnesium	Figs, lemons, grapefruit, yellow corn, almonds, nuts, seeds, dark green vegetables, apples
Manganese	Nuts, green leafy vegetables, peas, beets, egg yolk, whole-grain cereals
Molybdenum	Dark green leafy vegetables, whole grains, eggs, nuts, seeds
Phosphorus	Fish, poultry, meat, whole grains, eggs, nuts, seeds
Potassium	Citrus fruits, watercress, all green leafy vegetables, mint leaves, sunflower seeds, bananas, potatoes
Selenium	Wheat germ, bran, tunafish, onions, tomatoes, broccoli

MINERAL	BEST NATURAL SOURCES
Sodium	Salt, shellfish, carrots, beets, artichokes, dried beef, brains, kidney, bacon
Sulfur	Lean beef, dried beans, fish, eggs, cabbage
Vanadium	Fish
Water	Drinking water, juices, fruits and vegetables
Zinc	Round steak, lamb chops, pork loin, wheat germ, brewer's yeast, pumpkin seeds, eggs, nonfat dry milk, ground mustard

AMINO ACID	BEST NATURAL SOURCES
Tryptophan	Cottage cheese, milk, turkey, bananas, meat, dried dates, peanuts, all protein-rich foods
Phenylalanine	Soy products, bread stuffing, cottage cheese, dry skim milk, almonds, peanuts, lima beans, pumpkin seeds, sesame seeds, all protein-rich foods
Lysine	Fish, milk, lima beans, meat, cheese, yeast, eggs, soy products, all protein-rich foods
Arginine	Nuts, popcorn, carob, gelatin desserts, chocolate, brown rice, oatmeal, raisins, sunflower and sesame seeds, whole wheat bread, all protein-rich foods

129. Any Questions About Chapter 10?

If mayonnaise spoils so easily, why is it never refrigerated in the supermarket?

Mayonnaise doesn't spoil easily. In fact, unopened and unrefrigerated, it can remain fresh for at least 6 months, usually longer. Despite all the concern about food poisonings at picnics, mayonnaise is seldom if ever the cause. (It's too acidic for bacteria to grow in easily.) What happens is that when it is mixed with other foods, such as tunafish, eggs, and potatoes, it becomes a medium for bacterial growth.

The reason manufacturers recommend that it be refrigerated after opening is because when adding it to salads, most people will dip in for another spoonful, leaving some particles of food that can cause it to become a bacterial breeding ground. If kept refrigerated at temperatures of 40° F., it will remain harmless.

Salads mixed with mayonnaise should be kept cold until ready to eat. Leaving combinations like cooked chicken and mayonnaise out on a table for hours gives bacteria a field day and picnickers the trots.

Is it safe to refreeze frozen foods that have only partially thawed?

If the foods still contain ice crystals and have been held no longer than 1 or 2 days at refrigerator temperatures after thawing, they're generally safe to refreeze. (Thawed ice cream is an exception; it should not be refrozen.) As a rule, if a partially thawed food is safe to eat it's safe to refreeze. On the other hand, if there are any off-odors or -colors, the food should definitely not be refrozen—or eaten.

You must keep in mind, though, that refreezing reduces nutritional quality, particularly of fruits, vegetables, and prepared foods. Meats suffer less quality reduction. In all cases, it's best to use refrozen foods as soon as possible to get the most nutritional value from them.

Does olive oil have to be refrigerated, and if so how long should it be kept?

Olive oil keeps longer than any other edible oil. Refrigerating is not necessary, but it is not harmful either. What happens, though, is that the oil becomes cloudy and thick if refrigerated, which tends to make people think it has gone bad. It hasn't, and when left at room temperature it will regain its clarity and have lost none of its healthful properties. Olive oil stored in airtight containers in a cool, dark place, away from light, can last from 6 months to a year. Of course, if at any point it begins to smell odd, or change from its original green-goldish color, something is amiss and you'd be wise to throw it out.

When I was recovering from a nasty case of food poisoning, my doctor prescribed carrot soup. I was surprised. Has chicken soup been nutritionally usurped for some reason?

Not at all. Chicken soup is, and probably always will be, "Jewish penicillin" because of its natural antibiotic properties. But when recovering from dehydration caused by diarrhea, which you undoubtedly were, sodium and potassium are the two electrolytes most needed returned in proper balance. And carrot soup has them—in the correct proportions. According to Dr. Jan Soule, the Portland, Oregon, pediatrician who dished out the information to the medical community as well as to his patients, carrot soup is the best rehydrator.

Bouillon and canned soups have far too much sodium, and juices, although high in potassium, haven't a balanced amount of sodium. Herb teas can replace lost water but not electrolytes, and caffeinated beverages can *promote* dehydration. The soup can be made in a jiffy by combining equal amounts of water and commercial strained baby carrots (which have salt in them) and bringing the mixture to a boil.

11
FOODS FOR THOUGHT

130. The Diet-Disease Connection

The evidence linking diet to cancer, heart disease, diabetes, infertility, depression, and numerous other ailments is becoming stronger and stronger. Researchers are finding that overconsumption of foods high in fats and additives—unchecked by those high in fiber, anticarcinogens, and essential nutrients—can cause diseases that are far easier to prevent than cure.

This does not mean that any one diet, or particular food or supplement regimen, is the answer. Despite all the books and articles you might have read or heard about, *no diet can guarantee protection against illness*. But learning what foods have been shown to contribute to certain illnesses, avoiding or limiting their consumption, and counteracting their risks with alternative health-boosting foods can provide you with the best chance for a longer and healthier life.

131. Cancer Brewers

The National Academy of Sciences, National Cancer Institute, and American Cancer Society recommend that no more than 20 to 30 percent of the calories in your diet come from fat. Individuals whose diets contain over 40 percent fat, saturated as well as unsaturated, are more likely to develop colon, breast, and prostate cancers.

The following percentages of calories from fat, compiled by the Center for Science in the Public Interest, are given here to alert you to frequently eaten foods that you might want to change your mind about eating large quantities of frequently.

> The greater a food's fat content, the less often—and less of it—you should be eating.

For example, 2 tablespoons of mayonnaise have only 200 calories, but because 100 percent of those calories are fat, those 2 tablespoons equal 20 percent of your daily calorie intake, in effect *half* of what is considered a safe daily fat allotment. (If you're not up to dividing the number of calories in your food portions by their fat percentages, see section 89.)

FOOD	CALORIES FROM FAT
Butter, margarine, mayonnaise, oils	100%
Coconut	92%
Cream cheese	90%
Avocado	86%
Beef franks, bologna	80%
Peanut butter	76%
Cheddar cheese	74%
Chicken franks	68%
Swiss cheese	66%
Ground beef (lean)	65%
Eggs, potato chips	63%
Croissant (Pepperidge Farm)	59%
Mozzarella cheese (part skim), chicken breast (Kentucky Fried), milk chocolate candy bars	56%
Old-fashioned doughnuts (Hostess), Big Mac (McDonald's)	53%
Ricotta cheese (part skim), tofu, Fillet-O-Fish (McDonald's)	52%
Pork chop (lean), hamburger (Wendy's)	50%
Whole milk (4% fat)	49%

Food	Calories From Fat
Vanilla ice cream	48%
French fries	47%
Stouffer's entrees (average)	46%
Le Menu and Armour Dinner Classics (average), lamb (rib chop), veal (round)	45%
Chicken (dark, w/out skin)	43%
Apple pie (Morton's)	40%
Cottage cheese (4% fat)	39%
Cheese pizza (Pizza Hut, plain)	38%
Low-fat milk (2%), hamburger (McDonald's)	35%
Granola cereals	32–42%
Round steak (lean)	29%
Chicken (light, w/out skin)	24%
Low-fat milk (1%)	23%
Yogurt (low-fat, plain)	22%
Lean Cuisine meals (average)	21%

OTHER EDIBLE CANCER CONCERNS

• Food additives, particularly BHA, BHT, Food Dyes Red No. 3, Blue No. 2, Green No. 3 and Citrus Red No. 2, propyl gallate, and sodium nitrite.

• Coffee, regular or decaffeinated (implicated in bladder and pancreatic cancers).

• Liver and high-fat meat (contaminants accumulate in an animal's liver and fat cells).

• Certain high-fat fish, such as bluefish, striped bass, lake trout, and mackerel; and bottom-feeding fish, such as carp, which are more likely than others to contain high levels of contaminants.

• Alcohol (found to cause liver cancer and contribute to cancers of the mouth, throat, larynx and esophagus, particularly among smokers).

132. Foods That Can Fight Back

Foods high in vitamins A, C, E, selenium, and fiber (see section 128) have been found to help in the prevention of cancer. Eating three or more ½-cup servings of vegetables, particularly cruciferous vegetables containing indoles and isothiocyanates (substances that have been found to reduce the number of tumors in mice treated with carcinogens) is highly recommended.

Cruciferous vegetables that have been found to contain indoles and isothiocyanates are broccoli, brussels sprouts, cabbage, and cauliflower. Other cruciferous vegetables that are presumed to contain indoles and isothiocyanates, include bok choy, collards, kale, kohlrabi, mustard greens, rutabaga, and turnips.

133. Food Mood Swingers

There's little doubt that what we eat affects how we feel. In fact, numerous experiments have proven that many symptoms of mental illness can be switched off and on by changing diet and altering nutrient levels in the body.

Vitamin B_1 (thiamine)	Large amounts have been found to tranquilize anxious individuals and alleviate depression.
Vitamin B_2 (riboflavin)	Works synergistically with vitamins B_6, C, and niacin as a stress fighter. Insufficiencies are frequently found in individuals whose diets are too low in meat or dairy protein.
Vitamin B_6 (pyridoxine)	Insufficiencies can impair the function of the adrenal cortex and adversely affect production of natural antidepressants such as dopamine and norepinephrine.
Choline	One of the few nutrients able to penetrate the blood-brain barrier, which ordinarily protects the brain

Choline (cont'd.)	against variations in the daily diet, and go directly into brain cells to produce a chemical that aids memory. Dietary insufficiencies are frequently manifested by nervousness or twitching.
Pantothenic acid	A natural tension reliever when sufficient in diet.
Vitamin C (ascorbic acid)	Needed along with vitamin B_6 for the effective conversion of phenylalanine into mood-elevating norepinephrine.
Vitamin B_{12} (cobalamin)	Insufficient amounts can impair concentration, promote irritability, decrease energy, and increase anxiety.
Vitamin E (alpha-tocopherol)	Important for supplying adequate oxygen to brain cells.
Folic acid (folacin)	Deficiencies have been found to be contributing factors in mental illness.
Zinc	Promotes mental alertness and aids in proper brain function; deficiencies have frequently been found in schizophrenics.
Magnesium	Necessary for healthy nerve functioning; known as the anti-stress mineral.
Niacin	Lack of this B-complex vitamin can bring about negative personality changes.
Calcium	Alleviates tension, irritability, and promotes relaxation.

Tyrosine	An amino acid that releases a substance called catecholamine which, in turn, increases the production of the antidepressants dopamine and norepinephrine.
Tryptophan	An amino acid that functions synergistically with vitamin B$_6$, niacin, and magnesium to synthesize serotonin, a natural tranquilizer. (The availability of tryptophan and tyrosine in the brain is a major factor in determining the rate at which vital neurotransmitters are produced; within one hour after a meal moods can change according to the rise and fall of these two amino acids in the blood.)
Phenylalanine	An essential amino acid (found in cheese, meat, milk, and eggs) necessary for the manufacture and release of the brain's antidepressants dopamine and norepinephrine.

134. Eating Your Way to Depression

The quickest way to ruin your day is by eating the wrong foods. Refined sugars and carbohydrates, such as those in cakes, cookies, potato chips, pretzels, candy bars, sugared cereals, and junk foods, deplete your body of mood-regulating nutrients. Moreover, they play Ping-Pong with your glucose levels to the point of promoting antisocial, aggressive, and often violent behavior. (It has been found that 75 percent of all criminals have abnormal glucose levels.)

• Children and adolescents on high-sugar, refined carbohydrate diets have been found to undergo personality changes.

• Regular consumption of processed luncheon meats (bologna, hot dogs, ham, etc.) or convenience foods with artificial colorings and other additives can deplete not only essential stress-fighting B vitamins and zinc, but cause allergic reactions as well. (Instead of the usual ones, such as rashes or stomach upsets, artificial colorings and additives can, particularly in the case of children, cause a chemical reaction in the brain that's manifested by a sudden outburst of delinquent behavior.)

• If you are allergic to gluten, consuming products containing wheat, oats, rye, barley, or vegetables such as beans, cabbage, turnips, dried peas, and cucumbers can cause depression and fatigue. The same holds true if you are allergic to, and deliberately or inadvertently consume, dairy or citrus products.

• Chocolate, cocoa, and all caffeine-containing beverages (see section 47) can inhibit the proper assimilation of calcium and deplete the body of B-complex vitamins and zinc.

• Alcohol from wine, beer, spirits, or cough syrups can rob the body of vitamins B_1, B_2, choline, niacin, folic acid, and magnesium.

135. Depression and Stress Antidotes

APPETIZING UPPERS

Whole wheat products, brewer's yeast, wheat germ, fish, eggs, peanuts, the white meat of poultry, avocados, dates, figs, prunes, rice husks, oatmeal, bran, milk, green leafy vegetables, cantaloupe, cabbage, blackstrap molasses, lean meat, cheese, citrus fruits, berries, tomatoes, cauliflower, broccoli, brussel sprouts, ground mustard, potatoes, sweet potatoes, soybeans, sardines, salmon, walnuts, sunflower seeds, dried beans, dairy products, yellow corn, almonds, apples, lemons, grapefruit, peas, beets, bananas, lima beans, pumpkin and sesame seeds.

DELICIOUS DE-STRESSERS

• A glass of warm milk before bedtime is a soothing source of tryptophan, and can reduce anxiety and tension.

• Celery juice is a tangy and effective nerve unjangler for weight-conscious working men and women.

• A high-carbohydrate dinner can help you unwind and relax by raising the level of serotonin in the brain.

(NOTE: Because stress speeds up potassium loss, be sure to include bananas, potatoes, citrus fruits, and other potassium-rich foods in your daily diet.)

SUPPLEMENT SUGGESTIONS

• L-PA (L-phenylalanine) tabs (250–500 mg.), 3 daily, 1 hour before each meal. (When depression eases up, decrease to 1 tablet daily and then discontinue therapy.) If there is no improvement in 4 to 6 weeks, consult a nutritionally oriented physician (see section 143).
• Stress B complex with C, 1–3 times daily.
• Chelated calcium and magnesium, 3 tabs, 3 times daily. (The ratio should be twice as much calcium as magnesium.) Calcium gluconate is a vegetarian source and more potent than calcium lactate, which is a milk sugar derivative and easier to absorb. Doses over 2,000 mg. daily are *not* recommended unless specifically prescribed by a doctor.
• L-tryptophan, 500–667 mg., 1–3 times daily (with water, no protein).
• Propolis, 500 mg., take 15 to 20 minutes before each meal (preferably on an empty stomach), 1–3 times daily.

136. Foods Can Be Sex Sinkers

Just because you or your partner is not in the mood for love as often as you'd like to be doesn't necessarily mean that something is missing in your relationship. It could be missing from your diet.

A deficiency in zinc can cause a definite diminution of your sex drive. Vegetarians might make lousy lovers if they are consuming excessive amounts of calcium-rich greens and whole-grain cereals, breads, and bran, which contain phytic acid, because high intakes of these can prevent the absorption of zinc.

Drinking large amounts of coffee or other caffeinated beverages might keep you awake but put your sexual urges to sleep by inhibiting zinc absorption.

Eating frequent and hefty amounts of ice cream, beverages, candy, baked goods, gelatin desserts, and chewing gums that are artificially flavored with benzyl alcohol, butyl acetate, or benzaldehyde can produce central nervous system depression and reduce sexual urges and pleasures to memories.

If you are planning on having a family, avoid frequent consumption of shortenings, processed breakfast cereals, instant potatoes, snack foods, and others containing propyl gallate. This antioxidant has been implicated as a cause of reproductive failures.

Cocktails for two are romantic, but more than two cocktails can turn one enchanted evening into another depressing washout. Alcohol might increase sexual desire, but as many drinkers have discovered that's about all it increases.

137. Great Boosters for Better Sex

LOVE ENERGIZERS

Oysters, wheat germ, pumpkin and sunflower seeds, seafood, poultry, soybeans, melon, meat, avocados, green leafy vegetables, olive oil, eggs, whole-grain cereals, low-fat milk.

HERBS WITH SEX APPEAL

• Sarsaparilla has been used as a natural sexual stimulant for centuries. (The sarsaparilla plant has chemical substances with testosterone, progesterone, and cortisol activity, which probably accounts for its usefulness in increasing sexual appetites.) It is best when prepared by boiling an ounce of sarsaparilla root in a pint of water for half an hour—and most effective if wine-size glassfuls of it are drunk regularly.

• Damiana, an herb that's also called turnea, is known as a natural aphrodisiac. By simply pouring a cup of boiling water over a teaspoonful of the dried leaves (or ¼ teaspoonful of the ground leaf powder), it can be made into a tea. Drinking 1 to 4 cups daily—no more—has provided some tantalizing rewards for many who've tried it.

• Because of its normalizing effect on the body's metabolism, ginseng (see section 117) drunk as a tea or tonic can help reduce anxiety and heighten sexual stimulation.

SUPPLEMENT SUGGESTIONS

- Phenylalanine, 250–500 mg., daily
- Tyrosine, 250–500 mg., daily
- Chelated zinc, 15–50 mg., daily
- Vitamin A, 5,000–10,000 IU, daily 5 days a week (stop for 2 days)
- Vitamin C, 500–1,000 mg., 1–3 times daily
- Vitamin E (dry form), 200–800 IU, daily. (For postmenopausal women, mixed tocopherol vitamin E, 400 IU, daily is recommended.)
- Selenium, 50–100 mcg., daily
- Vitamin B complex, 50 mg., 1–3 times daily
- Optional for men: pumpkin seed oil (vitamin F), 3 capsules daily

138. Aging Accelerators

Everyone knows that eating the wrong foods in the wrong quantities can increase weight rapidly. But everyone doesn't know that it can also accelerate aging.

- Coffee, tea, cocoa, colas, and other caffeinated beverages are liquid youth-liquidators that dehydrate your skin and can cause premature wrinkling.
- There's no harm in an occasional glass of wine, but immoderate alcohol consumption can dehydrate skin, dilate blood vessels, foster spidery broken capillaries on the face, and add years to your looks while subtracting them from your life. (See section 76.)
- High-fat, high-protein, no- or low-carbohydrate diets—or any liquid, fad, or crash-reducing programs that produce a rapid weight loss by eliminating a category of nutrients—are dangerous potentiators of aging. Aside from causing skin to lose elasticity, and depleting nutrients necessary for the healthy regeneration of cells, they promote stress that can cause the release of actual aging chemicals in the body.
- Meat and milk, if consumed in large quantities, can inhibit the absorption of manganese, which is essential for the production of the anti-aging enzyme SOD (superoxide dismutase). SOD, which diminishes naturally as we age, fortifies the body against the ravages of free radicals, the destructive molecules that speed the aging process by destroying healthy cells and collagen.

• Processed foods that are high in refined carbohydrates and sugar can contribute to vision problems. (Nearsightedness and the amount of refined carbohydrates in the diet have been found to be almost directly proportional.)

• Excessive consumption of soft drinks, which are high in phosphorus, can deplete you of calcium and increase your chances of osteoporosis.

139. Help for Holding Back Advancing Years

YOUTH EXTENDERS

Wheat germ, bran, whole grains, spinach, asparagus, mushrooms, fish (especially sardines, salmon, and mackerel), chicken liver, oatmeal, onions, pumpkin seeds, brewer's yeast, dried beans, peas, prunes, green leafy vegetables, low-fat milk, olive oil.

VICTUALS FOR VITALITY

• A fish dish a day (or at least 5 times weekly) can help your body stay well supplied with the DNA-RNA nucleic acids that are essential for new cell growth.

• Eating substantial amounts of foods rich in PABA and folic acid (see section 128) can help retard the graying of hair—and possibly even return gray hair to its former color.

• An orange, a one-ounce slice of Cheddar cheese, and a glass of skim milk can supply half of your daily requirement for calcium; a pretty simple way to help keep your skin smooth, bones strong, and nerves on a healthy even keel.

SUGGESTED SUPPLEMENTS

• High-potency multiple vitamin with chelated minerals, A.M. and P.M., with meals

• Vitamin E with antioxidants (dry form for premenopausal women), 400 IU, 1–2 times daily

• Vitamin B complex, 50–100 mg., A.M. and P.M., with meals

• RNA–DNA, 100 mg. tablets, 1 daily for one month, then 2 daily for the next month, then 3 daily thereafter, 6 days a week
• SOD, 125 mcg., 1 daily for one month, then 2 daily the next month, then 3 daily thereafter, 6 days a week

140. Immunity Underminers

A healthy immune system is a stalwart army of white blood cells (called T-cells because they're controlled by the thymus gland) that is instructed where and when to attack and what antibodies their cofighters (called B-cells because they're made in the bone marrow) should produce. As you get older your thymus gland decreases in power and size, becomes a less effective commander of your defense brigade, and if not supplied with the right nutritional reinforcements, will let you down—the hard way.

Highly allergenic foods, such as shellfish, chocolate, and eggs, can cause the immune systems of susceptible individuals to create excessive antibodies when none are needed, resulting in a variety of discomforting and potentially dangerous symptoms.

• Frequent consumption of foods containing artificial flavors, colors, MSG, and other additives can stress the immune system, diminishing its effectiveness in protecting you from numerous illnesses and infections.
• Indulging in refined carbohydrates (cakes, cookies, junk food, etc.), caffeine, and alcohol can make you more vulnerable to infection and illness by depleting essential immune system nutrients.
• Irradiated foods, eaten on a regular basis, may impair bone marrow and adversely affect the immune system's production of B-cells.

141. Boosting Your Body's Defenses

THE NATURAL ''RAMBOS''

Carrots, fish (sardines, salmon, mackerel), skim milk, citrus fruits, green leafy vegetables, wheat germ, whole grains, bran, soybeans, broccoli, brussels sprouts, eggs, sesame seeds, brown rice, nuts, onions, pumpkin seeds, ground mustard, brewer's yeast, propolis, papaya.

THE RIGHT FUEL

• A diet low in fat and high in complex carbohydrates, especially those that are rich in fiber.
• Evening primrose oil, an herb whose active ingredient is gamma linoleic acid (GLA), can help in the production of hormonelike compounds called prostaglandins—which are vital to the immune system.
• Propolis, a resinlike material found in leaf buds and the bark of trees and collected by bees whose enzymes convert it into pollen, is a thymus gland stimulator and natural immune system enhancer.

SUPPLEMENT SUGGESTIONS

• Vitamin A, 10,000–25,000 IU daily, 5 days a week (stop for 2 days)
• Vitamin C, 1,000 mg., 1–3 times daily
• Vitamin E (dry form), 200–400 IU, 1–3 times daily
• Arginine, 2,000 mg. daily (taken with water, no protein, and on an empty stomach)
• Ornithine, 2,000 mg. daily (taken with water, no protein, and on an empty stomach)
• Cysteine, 1 daily with vitamin C (3 times as much vitamin C as cysteine)
• Selenium, 50–100 mcg. daily
• Zinc, chelated, 15–50 mg., 1–3 times daily
• Propolis, 500 mg., 1–3 times daily

142. Any Questions About Chapter 11?

I'm forty years old and my face still breaks out. I am a vegetarian, and I don't drink, smoke, or eat junk food. I eat only natural foods, lots of grains, and I can't imagine what in my diet is causing this.

It could be any of a number of things. It could even *be* a number of things—hormonal changes, allergic reaction, stress, and so on—but if it is diet-related, I'd suspect it is being caused by some androgenic (rich in male hormones) food. You might try keeping away from peanuts, peanut oil, wheat germ oil, and brewer's yeast for a while and see if your skin clears up. The amount of male hormones in these foods is small, but for anyone with a latent skin or hair problem, it's enough to cause trouble.

I've been on a very healthy and successful diet for the past 4 months (high-fiber, low-fat) and have lost 32 pounds. I feel fine, except for the fact that I haven't menstruated since I began dieting. I take a supplement daily, eat no junk food at all, and eat salad twice a day. My gynecologist found nothing wrong with me. What could I be missing?

My guess would be calories. The physical stress of losing more than 30 pounds (or as much as 15 percent of your body weight) in a relatively short time can suppress production of hypothalamic and pituitary hormones that are essential to the menstrual cycle. If you are exercising, you might be overdoing it. Keep in mind that diets providing fewer than 1,200 calories daily can cause problems and should not be undertaken without the supervision of a doctor.

My advice would be to eat 300 to 500 more calories daily and ease up on your workouts. I'd also suggest that you take, along with your vitamin supplement, a multiple chelated mineral tablet with at least 500 mg. of calcium and 250 mg. of magnesium (that also contains manganese, zinc, iron, selenium, chromium, copper, iodine, and potassium), vitamin C, 500–1,000 mg., and vitamin E, 200 IU (one that also contains selenium, chromium, copper, iodine, and potassium) with breakfast and dinner 6 days a week. By taking your supplements only 6 days a week and resting on the seventh, you don't have to worry about a buildup of fat-soluble vitamins in your system. If you don't start menstruating within 4 weeks, it's time for another visit to a gynecologist.

I've been told that there's an herb now on the market that can help cure impotence. Do you know anything about it?

I believe you're referring to yohimbine, an alkaloid (organic, nitrogen-containing compound) derived from the bark of tropical Rubiaceae trees, that is currently being used to treat certain types of erectile impotence. It's available without a prescription in homeopathic doses and herbal preparations at health food stores. Higher, therapeutic doses require a prescription and should not be taken without specific medical instructions. Yohimbine can produce stimulating effects resembling those caused by epinephrine, as well as hypotension, and might be contraindicated for certain individuals. As appealing as its aphrodisiac qualities are, I strongly suggest you check with your physician, or a nutritionally oriented doctor, before taking yohimbine on a regular basis.

12
MAY I HELP YOU?

143. How to Locate a Nutritionally Oriented Doctor

If you would like to consult a nutritionally oriented physician but don't know any in your area, the following organizations can help you find one. You should specify that you're seeking a Board certified physician—if such is the case—as not all nutritional health professionals are M.D.s. It should be understood that no endorsement or other opinion of any practitioner contacted through these services (or such practitioner's diagnoses, treatments, or credentials) is implied or should be inferred. As a courtesy, please be sure to enclose a stamped, self-addressed envelope with all queries.

American Academy of Medical
  Preventics
6151 West Century Blvd., Suite
  1114
Los Angeles, CA 90045
(213) 645-5350

American Holistic Medical
  Association
6932 Little River Turnpike
Annandale, VA 22003

American Holistic Nurses Association
Box 116
Telluride, CO 81435

Association for the Promotion of
  Herbal Healing
2000 Center St., Suite 1475
Berkeley, CA 94704

Consulting Nutritionists
3150 E. 41st Street
Tulsa, OK 74135

Consulting Nutritionists in Private
Practice
P.O. Box 345
Cold Springs, NY 10515

Heal (Human Ecology Action
League)
P.O. Box 1369
Evanston, IL 60204

Health Associates
1990 Broadway, Suite 1206
New York, NY 10023
(212) 307-1399

Hippocrates Health Institute
25 Exeter Street
Boston, MA 02116

Huxley Institute for Biosocial
Research
900 N. Federal Highway, Suite 330
Boca Raton, FL 33432

International Academy of Holistic
Health & Medicine
218 Avenue B
Redondo Beach, CA 90277
(213) 540-0564

International Academy of
Metabiology, Inc.
P.O. Box 15157
Las Cruces, NM 88001

International Academy of Preventive
Medicine
34 Corporate Woods, Suite 469
Overland Park, KS 66210

International College of Applied
Nutrition
P.O. Box 386
La Habra, CA 90631
(818) 697-4576

International Foundation for
Homeopathy
1141 N.W. Market
Seattle, WA 98107
(206) 789-7237

National Association of Naturopathic
Physicians
2613 N. Stevens
Tacoma, WA 98407
(206) 789-7237

National Center for Homeopathy
1500 Massachusetts Ave. N.W., Suite
163
Washington, DC 20005
(202) 223-6182

National Health Federation
211 W. Foothill Blvd.
Monrovia, CA 91016
(818) 357-2181

Natural Hygiene Society
698 Brooklawn Ave.
Bridgeport, CT 06604

Northwest Academy of Preventive
Medicine
15615 Bellevue-Redmont Road,
Suite E
Bellevue, WA 98008

Nutrition for Optimal Health
Association
P.O. Box 380
Winnetka, IL 60093

Prevention Magazine Readers'
Service
Emmaus, PA 18049

Society for Clinical Ecology
2005 Franklin St., Suite 490
Denver, CO 80205

The Huxley Institute
210 E. 31st Street
New York, NY 10016
(Distributes information on both
orthomolecular psychiatry and
medicine.)

144. Finding Specialized Nutritional Help
Enclose a stamped, self-addressed envelope with all queries.

For alcoholism

Alcoholics Anonymous
P.O. Box 459
Grand Central Station
New York, NY 10163

For allergies

National Institute of Allergy
and Infectious Diseases
NIH, Dept. of Health and Human
Services
Bldg. 31, Room 7A32
Bethesda, MD 20205

For Alzheimer illnesses

Alzheimer's Disease and Related
Disorders Association
360 North Michigan Ave.
Suite 1102
Chicago, IL 60601

ALS Society of America
15300 Ventura Blvd.
Suite 315
Sherman Oaks, CA 91403

For arthritis

Arthritis Information
Clearinghouse
Box 34427
Bethesda, MD 20817

For breast-feeding   La Leche League, Intl., Inc.
  and pregnancy   9616 Minneapolis Ave.
                            Franklin Park, IL 60131

For cancer   Cancer Control Society
                            2043 North Berendo
                            Los Angeles, CA 90027

                            International Association of
                              Cancer Victors and
                              Friends, Inc.
                            7740 West Manchester Ave.,
                            Suite 1102
                            Playa del Rey, CA 90291

                            National Cancer Institute
                            NIH, Bldg. 31, Rm. 10A18
                            Bethesda, MD 20205

For cardiovascular disorders   Association for Cardiovascular
                              Therapy
                            P.O. Box 706
                            Bloomfield, CT 06002

                            Association of Heart Patients
                            P.O. Box 54305
                            Atlanta, GA 30308

                            The Stroke Foundation, Inc.
                            898 Park Avenue
                            New York, NY 10021

For communicative disorders   American Tinnitus Association
                            P.O. Box 5
                            Portland, OR 97207

                            Hearing and Tinnitus Help
                              Association
                            P.O. Box 97
                            Skillman, NJ 08558

For communicative
disorders (cont'd.)

National Council of Stutterers
P.O. Box 8171
Grand Rapids, MI 49508

For depression

Academy of Orthomolecular
    Psychiatry
P.O. Box 372
Manhasset, NY 11030

For diabetes

National Diabetic Information
    Clearinghouse
805 15th St. N.W., Rm. 500
Washington, DC 20005

For eating disorders

American Anorexia Nervosa
    Association, Inc.
133 Cedar Lane
Teaneck, NJ 07666

ANAD (National Association of
    Anorexia Nervosa and
    Associated Disorders)
Box 271
Highland Park, IL 60035
Hotline: (312) 831-3438

Center for the Study of
    Anorexia and Bulimia
1 West 91st Street
New York, NY 10024

Help Anorexia, Inc.
5143 Overland Avenue
Culver City, CA 90230

National Institute of
    Arthritis, Metabolism,
    and Digestive Diseases
NIH, Bldg. 31, Rm. 9A04
Bethesda, MD 20205

For hypoglycemia

National Hypoglycemia
   Association
P.O. Box 885
Ithaca, NY 14850

For pets

The American Veterinary
   Holistic Medical Assoc.
2214 Old Emmerton Rd.
Bel Air, MD 21014

For sleep disorders

Association for Sleep Disorders
   Center (ASDC)
Box 2604
Del Mar, CA 92014

For women

Coalition for the Medical
   Rights of Women
2845 24th Street
San Francisco, CA 94110

National Women's Health Network
224 7th St. S.E.
Washington, DC 20003

145. Free Calls for Fast Answers and Action

• For information about diet and cancer, the National Cancer Institute will answer any question they can. Just call 1-800-4-CANCER.

• For information on water contaminants, waste disposal sites, and dangerous chemicals, the Environmental Protection Agency's hotline is 1-800-424-9065.

• For product recall information, the Consumer Product Safety Commission's hotline is 1-800-492-8363.

• To register complaints about food fraud, waste, or abuse, call the Department of Agriculture's hotline, 1-800-424-9121.

• For answers to questions about the safety of your drinking water, you can phone Water Test Corp. toll free, 1-800-426-8378.

• For information on health, safety, ingredients, and nutritive value of baby foods, call Beech-Nut's Nutrition hotline, 1-800-523-6633.

• If you want to know more about herbs, where to obtain them, and have questions about their safety and usage, you can call Penn Herb (1-800-523-9971), Herbal Pathways (1-800-631-3575), Green Mountain Herbs (1-800-525-2696), or Foodscience Corporation (1-800-451-5190) for the answers.

• Vegetarians who would like to learn more ways to use meat analogs in their diet can call Morningstar Farms, a division of Miles Laboratories, for recipes and suppliers. The toll-free number is 1-800-243-4143.

GETTING MORE FAST INFORMATION AND ACTION FOR THE PRICE OF A PHONE CALL

• Questions on any aspect of human nutrition and food composition and interaction can be answered quickly by the Human Nutrition Center (202) 447-5121, or the Food and Nutrition Information and Education Resources Center (301) 344-3719.

• Problems or questions about nutritional labeling of meat and poultry can be cleared up by phoning the USDA division of standards and labeling at (202) 447-7620. To register complaints, the number is (301) 344-2003.

• If you have any questions concerning the use or safety of any foods or drugs now being marketed, call the FDA office of Consumer Communications at (301) 443-3170.

• To report problem products and register complaints, you can telephone one of the FDA's regional offices, or phone (301) 443-1240. If it is an emergency, call their 24-hour answering service at (202) 737-0448.

146. Any Questions About Chapter 12?

Are there any computer services that give updates and advice on foods, additives, and nutrition in general?

There are quite a few. Nutri-line (7422 Mount Joy Drive, Huntington Beach, CA 92648, [714] 848-1202) is one. It's a computerized reference service that has the latest information, from reliable sources, available and easily accessible. There are also several software programs being sold that can provide you with data bases for solving a wide variety of nutritional problems, and games that employ nutritional principles. Unfortunately, most are limited in their scope and practicality, which is why I am preparing *The Vitamin Bible* for release as a total health and nutrition computer program, with flexible and multifaceted uses, right now.

How can I become more active in effecting changes in food malpractices such as misleading advertising, and the use of unsafe pesticides and additives?

You can begin by writing complaints (and getting your friends to do the same) to the Food and Drug Administration, Department of Health and Human Services, 5600 Fishers Lane (HFO-410), Room 1362, Rockville, MD 20857. Informing your state attorney general of any product with misleading advertising, and expressing disapproval of EPA and FDA policies in letters to government representatives, can often be more effective than most people think.

If you want to really get involved in forcing our food suppliers to clean up their act, I'd suggest contacting the Center for Science in the Public Interest (CSPI), a nonprofit public interest organization that publishes *Nutrition Action Healthletter* ten times a year. They have helped organize and support numerous effective lobbying groups, such as Americans for Safe Foods and the National Coalition Against the Misuse of Pesticides (both of which are organizing and expanding local chapters across the nation). For membership and other information, write or phone:

The Center for Science in the Public Interest (CSPI)
1501 16th St. N.W.
Washington, DC 20036
(202) 332-9110

Afterword

I hope I've been able to provide enough information to enable you to minimize the risks of foods and maximize their potential for providing you with health, longevity, and happiness at every meal.

With that in mind, I leave you with these parting morsels:

- Heptachlor, a carcinogenic grain pesticide banned in 1983, is still showing up in mother's breast milk.
- Every unwanted nutrient in the American diet is supplied in large doses by white bread, rolls, and crackers, because they're eaten so frequently.
- Some of us may live to eat, but all of us must eat to live—and what we eat *can* change our lives.

To your health!

EARL L. MINDELL, R.PH., PH.D

Beverly Hills, California
September, 1986

216

Glossary

Absorption: The process by which nutrients are passed into the bloodstream.

Acetate: A derivative of acetic acid.

Acetic acid: Used as a synthetic flavoring agent, one of the first food additives (vinegar is approximately 4 to 6 percent acetic acid); it is found naturally in cheese, coffee, grapes, peaches, raspberries, and strawberries. Generally Recognized As Safe (GRAS) when used only in packaging.

Acetone: A colorless solvent for fat, oils, and waxes that is obtained by fermentation (inhalation can irritate lungs, and large amounts have a narcotic effect).

Acid: A water-soluble substance with a sour taste.

Addiction: Compulsive use of habit-forming drugs.

Adrenal gland: A triangular-shaped gland near each kidney that synthesizes and stores dopamine, norepinephrine, and epinephrine.

Alkali: An acid-neutralizing substance (sodium bicarbonate is an alkali used for excess acidity in foods).

Allergen: A substance that causes an allergy.

Allergy: Abnormal sensitivity to any substance.

Amenorrhea: Absence or suppression of menstruation.

Amino acid chelates: Chelated minerals that have been produced by many of the same processes nature uses to chelate minerals in the body; in the digestive tract, nature surrounds the elemental minerals with amino acid, permitting them to be absorbed into the bloodstream.

217

Amino acids: The organic compounds from which proteins are constructed; there are twenty-two known amino acids, but only nine are indispensable nutrients for man—histidine, isoleucine, leucine, lysine, total S-containing amino acids, total aromatic amino acids, threonine, tryptophan, and valine—and must be obtained from food.

Analgesic: Drug used to relieve pain.

Anemia: Reduction in normal amount of red blood cells.

Anorectic: Having no appetite.

Anorexia nervosa: A symptom of mental disturbance that causes loss of appetite for food and compulsive dieting.

Antibiotic: Any of various substances that are effective in inhibiting or destroying bacteria.

Anticoagulant: Something that delays or prevents blood clotting; blood thinner.

Antidyskinetics: Drugs used in the treatment of Parkinson's disease.

Antiemetic: Remedy to prevent vomiting.

Antigen: Any substance not normally present in the body that stimulates the body to produce antibodies.

Antihistamine: A drug used to reduce effects associated with colds and allergies.

Antineoplastics: Drugs that prevent the growth and development of malignant cells.

Antioxidant: A substance that can protect another substance from oxidation; added to foods to keep oxygen from changing the food's color.

Antispasmodic: A drug used to relieve cramping and spasms of the stomach, intestines, and bladder.

Antitoxin: An antibody formed in response to—and capable of—neutralizing a poison of biologic origin.

Aphrodisiac: An agent that produces sexual desire.

Apnea: Temporary cessation of breathing, usually during sleep.

Arthritis: Inflammation of joints.

Assimilation: The process whereby nutrients are used by the body and changed into living tissue.

Asthma: Condition of lungs characterized by a decrease in diameter of some air passages; a spasm of the bronchial tubes or swelling of their mucous membranes.

Ataxia: Loss of coordinated movement.

Avidin: A protein in egg white capable of inactivating biotin.

Bariatrician: A weight-control doctor.

BATF: Bureau of Alcohol, Tobacco, and Firearms.

BHA: Butylated hydroxyanisole; a preservative and antioxidant used in many products; insoluble in water; can be toxic to the kidneys.

BHT: Butylated hydroxytoluene; a solid, white crystalline antioxidant used to retard spoilage of many foods; can be more toxic to the kidneys than its nearly identical chemical cousin, BHA.

Bioflavonoids: Usually from orange and lemon rinds, these citrus-flavored compounds needed to maintain healthy blood-vessel walls are widely available in plants, citrus fruits, and rose hips; known as vitamin P-complex.

Calciferol: A colorless, odorless crystalline material that is insoluble in water, soluble in fats; a synthetic form of vitamin D made by irradiating ergosterol with ultraviolet light.

Calcium gluconate: An organic form of calcium.

Carcinogen: A cancer-causing substance.

Cardiac arrhythmia: Irregular heart action caused by disturbances in the discharge of cardiac impulses.

Cardiovascular: Pertaining to heart and blood vessels.

Carotene: An orange-yellow pigment in many plants that can be converted into vitamin A in the body.

Casein: The protein in milk that has become the standard by which protein quality is measured.

Catalyst: A substance that modifies, especially increases, the rate of chemical reaction without being consumed or changed in the process.

Cataract: Clouding of the lens of the eye which prevents clear vision.

Cellulose: A fibrous, nondigestible carbohydrate; aids in intestinal elimination; provides no nutrient value.

Chelation: A process by which mineral substances are changed into easily digestible form.

Chronic: Of long duration; continuing; constant.

Cirrhosis: A chronic liver disease characterized by dense or hardened connective tissue, degenerative changes, or alteration in structure.

CNS: Central nervous system.

Coenzyme: The major portion, though nonprotein part, of an enzyme; usually a B vitamin.

Colitis: Inflammation of the large intestine.

Collagen: The primary organic constituent of bone, cartilage, and connective tissue (becomes gelatin through boiling).

Congenital: Condition existing at birth, not hereditary.

Corticosterone: An adrenal cortex hormone that influences the metabolism of carbohydrates, potassium, and sodium; essential for normal absorption of glucose.

Cortisone: An adrenal gland hormone; also used as an anti-inflammatory agent.

CPR: Cardiopulmonary resuscitation.

Dehydration: A condition resulting from an excessive loss of water from the body.

Dermatitis: An inflammation of the skin; a rash.

Desiccated: Dried; preserved by removing moisture.

Dicalcium phosphate: A filler used in pills that is derived from purified mineral rocks and is an excellent source of calcium and phosphorus.

Diluents: Fillers; inert material added to tablets to increase their bulk in order to make them a practical size for compression.

Diuretic: Increases the flow of urine from the body.

DNA: Deoxyribonucleic acid; the nucleic acid in chromosomes that is part of the chemical basis for hereditary characteristics.

Dyspepsia: Indigestion.

EDB: Ethylene dibromide; a carcinogenic pesticide used to fumigate grain.

Edema: Excessive accumulation of tissue fluid.

Endogenous: Produced from within the body.

Enteritis: Inflammation of the intestines, particularly the small intestines.

Enzyme: A protein substance found in living cells that brings about chemical changes; necessary for digestion of food.

EPA: Environmental Protection Agency.

Epidermis: The outer layer of skin.

Epilepsy: Convulsive disorder.

Estrogens: Female sex hormones.

Excipient: Any inert substance used as a dilutant or vehicle for a drug.

Exogenous: Derived or developed from external causes.

FBD: Fibrocystic breast disease, a common condition in which often painful, noncancerous cysts or lumps develop in the breast.

FDA: Food and Drug Administration.

Fibrin: An insoluble protein that forms the necessary fibrous network in the coagulation of blood.

Free radicals: Highly reactive chemical fragments that can produce an irritation of artery walls, start the arteriosclerotic process if vitamin E is not present; generally harmful.

Fructose: A natural sugar occurring in fruits and honey; often used as a preservative for foodstuffs.

Glucose: Blood sugar; a product of the body's assimilation of carbohydrates and a major source of energy.

Glutamic acid: An amino acid present in all complete proteins; usually manufactured from vegetable protein; used as a salt substitute and a flavor-intensifying agent; may affect CNS.

Glutamine: An amino acid that constitutes, with glucose, the major nourishment used by the nervous system.

Gluten: A mixture of two proteins—gliadin and glutenin—present in wheat, rye, oats, and barley.

Glycogen: The body's chief storage carbohydrate, primarily in the liver.

Gout: Upset in metabolism of uric acid, causing inflammation of joints, particularly in the knee or foot.

GRAS: Generally Recognized As Safe; a list established by Congress to cover substances added to food.

Half-life: The time it takes for half the amount of a drug to be metabolized or inactivated by the body (disappear from the bloodstream); an important consideration for determining the amount and frequency of drug dosage.

Hepatitis: Inflammation of the liver.

Hesperidin: Part of the C-complex.

HFCS: High fructose corn syrup.

Holistic treatment: Treatment of the whole person.

Homeostasis: The body's physiological equilibrium.

Hormone: A substance formed in endocrine organs and transported by body fluids to activate other specifically receptive organs.

HPP: Hydrolyzed plant protein, generally made from soybean or peanut meals. (See HVP.)

Humectant: A substance that is used to preserve the moisture content of materials.

HVP: Hydrolyzed vegetable protein, generally obtained from protein recovered from the wet milling of grains such as wheat and corn. Sometimes identified on labels as *hydrolyzed cereal* solids; components contain glutamic acid.

Hydrochloric acid: A normally acidic part of the body's gastric juice.

Hydrolyzed: Put into water-soluble form.

Hydrolyzed protein chelate: Water-soluble and chelated for easy assimilation.

Hypertension: High blood pressure.

Hypervitaminosis: A condition caused by an excessive ingestion of vitamins.

Hypoglycemia: Low blood sugar.

Hypotension: Low blood pressure.

Hypovitaminosis: A deficiency disease owing to an absence of vitamins in the diet.

Idiopathic: Of a condition whose causes are not yet known.

Immune: Protected against disease.

Infectious: Likely to be transmitted by infection.

Inflammation: Changes that occur in living tissues when invaded by germs; swelling, pain, heat.

Insulin: The hormone secreted by the pancreas that regulates the metabolism of sugar in the body.

IU: International Units.

Jaundice: Increase in bile pigment in blood, causing yellow tinge to skin, membranes, and eyes; can be caused by disease of the liver, gallbladder, bile system, or blood.

Lactating: Producing milk.

Lactation: Secretion of milk by breasts.

LAL: Lysinoalanine, a substance formed by the heating of casein, along with an alkali-treating process, that is suspected of causing kidney damage.

Laxative: A substance that stimulates evacuation of the bowels.

Linoleic acid: One of the polyunsaturated fats, a constituent of lecithin; known as vitamin F; indispensable for life; must be obtained from foods.

Lipid: A fat or fatty substance.

Lipofuscin: Age pigment in cells.

Lipotropic: Preventing abnormal or excessive accumulation of fat in the liver.

MAO inhibitors: Abbreviation for monoamine oxidase inhibitors; a group of antidepressants that promote an elevation of levels of amine messengers in the emotional regions of the brain.

Megavitamin therapy: Treatment of illness with massive amounts of vitamins.

Menopause: Age at which normal cessation of monthly period occurs, usually between forty-five and fifty.

Metabolize: To undergo change by physical and chemical processes.

Narcotic: A central nervous system depressant that, in moderate doses, relieves pain and produces sleep; in large doses it can produce unconsciousness or even death; can be addicting.

Nausea: Stomach discomfort with the feeling of a need to vomit.

Neuron: Nerve cell.

Neurotransmitter: A chemical that transports messages between neurons in the brain.

Nitrites: Substances used as fixatives in cured meats; can combine with natural stomach and food chemicals to cause dangerous cancer-causing agents called nitrosamines.

Obesity: Excessive stoutness.

Ophthalmic: Pertaining to eyes.

Orthomolecular: The right molecule used for the right treatment; doctors who practice preventive medicine and use vitamin therapies are known as orthomolecular physicians.

OSHA: Occupational Safety and Health Administration.

Osteoporosis: A condition characterized by porous (softening or increasingly brittle) bones.

Oxalates: Organic chemicals found in certain foods, especially spinach, which can combine with calcium to form calcium oxalate, an insoluble chemical the body cannot use.

PABA: Para-aminobenzoic acid; a member of the B-complex.

Palmitate: Water-solubilized vitamin A.

Parasite: Any animal or plant that lives inside or on the body of another animal or plant.

PCBs: Polychlorinated bipheyls; toxic industrial waste contaminants.

Peptic: Pertaining to the digestive tract.

PH: Degree of acidity or alkalinity of a substance.

Photosensitivity: Sensitivity to light.

PKU (phenylketonuria): A hereditary disease caused by the lack of an enzyme needed to convert an essential amino acid (phenylalanine) into a form usable by the body; can cause mental retardation unless detected early.

Polyunsaturated fats: Highly nonsaturated fats from vegetable sources; tend to lower blood cholesterol.

Predigested protein: Protein that has been processed for fast assimilation to go directly into the bloodstream.

Provitamin: A vitamin precursor; a chemical substance necessary to produce a vitamin.

Psoriasis: A skin condition characterized by silver-scaled red patches.

Psychosis: Type of insanity in which one almost completely loses touch with reality.

PUFA: Polyunsaturated fatty acid.

Radon: A naturally occurring form of radiation that seeps upward from the ground; carcinogenic.

RDA: Recommended Dietary Allowances as established by the Food and Nutrition Board, National Academy of Sciences, and National Research Council.

Rhinitis: Inflammation of the lining of the nose.

RNA: Ribonucleic acid.

Rose hips: A rich source of vitamin C; the nodule underneath the bud of a rose called a hip, in which the plant produces the vitamin C we extract.

Rutin: A substance extracted from buckwheat; part of the C-complex.

Saturated fatty acids: Usually solid at room temperature; higher proportions found in foods from animal sources; tend to raise blood cholesterol levels.

Sequestrant: A substance that absorbs ions and prevents changes that would affect the flavor, texture, and color of food; used for water softening.

Soporific: Producing sleep.

Steroid hormones: The sex hormones and hormones of the adrenal cortex.

Steroids: A family of cortisone-like medications; prescribed when adrenal glands do not produce enough of the hormone cortisone; also used for treatment of swellings, allergic reactions, and other conditions.

Sulfonamides: A group of sulfa drugs used to treat specific infections that are not responsive to other antibacterials.

Synergistic: The action of two or more substances to produce an effect that neither alone could accomplish.

Synthetic: Produced artificially.

Systemic: Pertaining to the whole body.

Tachycardia: Rapid beating of the heart coming on in sudden attacks.

Teratogen: Anything that causes the development of abnormalities in an embryo.

Tocopherols: The group of compounds (alpha, beta, delta, epsilon, eta, gamma, and zeta) that make vitamin E; obtained through the vacuum distillation of edible vegetable oils.

Topical: Applied externally.

Toxicity: The quality or condition of being poisonous, harmful, or destructive.

Toxin: An organic poison produced in living or dead organisms.

Triglycerides: Fatty substances in the blood.

Ulcer: Sore or lesion on skin surface or internal mucous membranes.

Unsaturated fatty acids: Most often liquid at room temperature; primarily found in vegetable fats.

USAN: United States Adopted Names Council; cosponsored by the American Pharmaceutical Association (APhA), American Medical Association (AMA), and United States Pharmacopia (USP) for the specific purpose of coining suitable, acceptable, nonproprietary names in the drug field.

U.S.RDA: United States Recommended Daily Allowances.

Vasodilator: A drug that dilates (widens) blood vessels.

Zein: Protein from corn.

Zyme: A fermenting substance.

Bibliography and Recommended Reading

To the nutritionists, pharmacists, doctors, scientists, therapists, dieticians, researchers, government agencies, and authors whose works in the field of health and nutrition proved indispensable to the scope and completion of this book, I owe an enormous debt of gratitude.

The list that follows is given to acknowledge my sincere and wholehearted appreciation to them, and to provide you with an opportunity for further reading in areas pertaining to your own particular interest or special medical and nutritional needs. Although some of the books are quite technical, those I've marked with asterisks are highly commended to all.

*Abrahamson, E. M., and Pezet, A. W. *Body, Mind and Sugar.* New York: Avon Books, 1977.

*Adams, Ruth, and Murray, Frank. *Minerals: Kill or Cure.* New York: Larchmont Books, 1976.

*Bennett, William, and Gurin, Joel. *The Dieter's Dilemma.* New York: Basic Books, 1982.

Berkow, Robert, ed. *The Merck Manual,* 14th ed. Rahway, NJ: Merck and Co., 1982.

*Brace, Edward R. *The Pediatric Guide to Drugs and Vitamins.* New York: Dell, 1982.

*Bricklin, Mark. *Practical Encyclopedia of Natural Healing.* Emmaus, PA: Rodale Press, 1976.

*Brody, Jane. *Jane Brody's Good Food Book: Living the High-Carbohydrate Way*. New York: Norton, 1985.

*_____ . *Jane Brody's Nutrition Book*. New York: Norton, 1981; Bantam, 1982.

*_____ . *The New York Times Guide to Personal Health*. New York: Times Books, 1982.

*Burns, David D. *Feeling Good, The New Mood Therapy*. New York: New American Library, 1980.

Clark, Matt, with Marianna Gosnell, Mary Hager, and Shawn Doherty. "The Calcium Craze," *Newsweek* (January 27, 1986).

Consumer Reports. "How Good Is Your Breakfast?" October 1986.

Consumer Reports, Editors of. *The Medicine Show*. Mount Vernon, NY: Consumers Union, 1981.

Cumulative Index for Journal of Applied Nutrition. La Habra, CA: International College of Applied Nutrition, 1947–76, 1976.

*de Bairacli Levy, Juliette. *Common Herbs for Natural Health*. New York: Schocken Books, 1974.

*Dufty, William. *Sugar Blues*. Philadelphia: Chilton Book Company, 1975.

*Edelstein, Barbara. *The Woman Doctor's Diet for Women*. New York: Prentice-Hall, 1977.

"Food Facts Talk Back," *Journal of the American Dietetic Association*, 1977.

*Frank, Benjamin S. *No-Aging Diet*. New York: Dial, 1976.

*Fredericks, Carlton. *Eating Right for You*. New York: Grosset and Dunlap, 1972.

*_____ . *Look Younger/Feel Healthier*. New York: Grosset and Dunlap, 1977.

*_____ . *Psycho Nutrients*. New York: Grosset and Dunlap, 1976.

*Freudenberger, Herbert J. *Burnout: The High Cost of High Achievement*. New York: Anchor Press, 1980.

*Gomez, Joan, and Gerch, Marvin J. *Dictionary of Symptoms*. New York: Bantam Books, 1972.

Goodhart, Robert S., and Shills, Maurice E. *Modern Nutrition in Health and Disease*, 5th ed. Philadelphia: Lea and Febiger, 1973.

*Gottlieb, Annie, and Sher, Barbara. *Wishcraft: How to Get What You Really Want*. New York: Ballantine, 1983.

*Graedon, Joe. *The People's Pharmacy,* vol 2. New York: Avon Books, 1980.

*Grosser, Arthur E. *The Cook Book Decoder, or Culinary Alchemy Explained.* New York and Toronto: Beaufort Books, 1981.

*Gutin, Bernard, with Kessler, Gail. *The High-Energy Factor.* New York: Random House, 1983.

*Hass, Robert. *Eat to Win: The Sports Nutrition Bible.* New York: Rawson Associates, 1984.

Howe, Phyllis S. *Basic Nutrition in Health and Disease,* 6th ed. Philadelphia: W. B. Saunders Co., 1976.

International College of Applied Nutrition. *Nutrition—Applied Personally.* La Habra, Ca, 1978.

Journal of the American Dietetic Association. "Vitamin-Mineral Safety, Toxicity, and Misuse," 1978.

*Kraus, Barbara. *The Barbara Kraus 1983 Sodium Guide to Brand Names and Basic Foods.* New York: Signet, 1983.

Krupp, M. A., and Chatton, M. J. *Current Medical Diagnosis and Treatment.* Los Altos, CA: Long Medical Publications, 1983.

*Kurtz, Irma. *Beds of Nails and Roses: A Guide to Your Emotions.* New York: Dodd, Mead & Co., 1983.

*Lansky, Vicki. *The Taming of the C.A.N.D.Y. Monster.* Wayzata, MN: Meadowbrook Press, 1978.

*Lesko, Matthew. *Information U.S.A.* New York: Viking Press, 1983.

*Linde, Shirley. *The Whole Health Catalog.* New York: Rawson Associates, 1977.

*Lipske, Michael, and Staff of the Center for Science in the Public Interest. *Chemical Additives in Booze.* Washington, DC: CSPI Books, 1982.

*London, Mel. *Breadwinners Too.* Emmaus, PA: Rodale Press, 1984.

*Lucas, Richard. *Nature's Medicines.* New York: Prentice-Hall, 1966.

*Lust, John. *The Herb Book.* New York: Bantam Books, 1974.

*Madders, Jane. *Stress and Relaxation.* New York: Arco, 1979.

*Martin, Alice A., and Tenenbaum, Frances. *Diet Against Disease.* Boston: Houghton Mifflin, 1980.

*Martin, Clement G. *Low Blood Sugar: The Hidden Menace of Hypoglycemia.* New York: Arco, 1976.

*Mayer, Jean. *A Diet for Living.* New York: David McKay, 1975.

Medical Economics. *Physician's Desk Reference,* 36th ed. Oradell, NJ: Medical Economics Company, 1982.

*Minear, Ralph E., M.D. *The Joy of Living Salt-Free*. New York: Macmillan, 1984.

National Dairy Council. *Nutrition Source Book*. Rosemont, IL: 1978.

National Nutrition Consortium, American Dietetic Association. *Nutrition Labeling: How It Can Work for You*. 1975.

National Nutrition Education Clearing House. *Nutrition Information Resources for the Whole Family*. 1978.

National Research Council. *Recommended Dietary Allowances*, 9th ed., rev. Washington, DC: National Academy of Sciences, 1980.

————. *Toxicants Occurring Naturally in Foods*, 2nd ed. Washington, DC: National Academy of Sciences, 1973.

*Newbold, H. L. *Dr. Newbold's Revolutionary New Discovery About Weight Loss*. New York: Rawson Associates, 1977.

*————. *Mega-Nutrients for Your Nerves*. New York: Peter H. Wyden, 1978.

Nutrition Almanac. New York: McGraw-Hill, 1979.

*Panos, Maesimund, and Heimlich, Jane. *Homeopathic Medicine at Home*. Los Angeles: J. P. Tarcher, 1980. Distributed by Houghton Mifflin Co., Boston.

*Passwater, Richard A. *Super Nutrition*. New York: Dial, 1975.

*Pauling, Linus. *Vitamin C and the Common Cold*. New York: Bantam Books, 1971.

*Pearson, Durk, and Shaw, Sandy. *Life Extension*. New York: Warner Books, 1982.

*Pomeranz, Virginia E., and Schultz, Dodi. *The Mothers' and Fathers' Medical Encyclopedia*. New York: New American Library, 1977.

*Pope, Carl. "Should Tap Water Be for Drinking?" *California Magazine* (September 1986).

*Pritikin, Nathan. *The Pritikin Permanent Weight-Loss Manual*. New York: Grosset and Dunlap, 1981.

Reader's Digest, Editors of. *Eat Better, Live Better*. Pleasantville, NY: Reader's Digest Association, 1982.

*Rodale, J. I. *The Encyclopedia of Common Diseases*. Emmaus, PA: Rodale Press, 1976.

Roe, Daphne A. *Handbook: Interactions of Selected Drugs and Nutrients in Patients*. Chicago: The American Dietetic Association, 1982.

*Seaman, Barbara, and Seaman, Gideon. *Women and the Crisis in Sex Hormones*. New York: Rawson Associates, 1977.

Thomas, Clayton I., ed. *Taber's Cyclopedic Medical Dictionary*, 14th ed. Philadelphia: F. A. Davis, 1982.

Underwood, Eric J. *Trace Elements in Human and Animal Nutrition*, 4th ed. New York: Academic Press, 1977.

U.S. Department of Agriculture. *Amino Acid Content of Food*, by M. L. Orr and B. K. Watt, 1957; rev. 1968.

U.S. Department of Agriculture, Consumer and Food Economics Institute, Agricultural Research Service. *Composition of Foods: Raw, Processed, Prepared*, by Bernice K. Watt and Annabel L. Merrill, 1975.

U.S. Department of Agriculture. *Energy Value of Foods: Basis and Derivation*, by Annabel L. Merrill and Bernice K. Watt, 1973.

U.S. Department of Agriculture. *Nutritive Value of American Foods*, by Catherine F. Adams, 1975.

The United States Pharmacopeial Convention. *The Physicians' and Pharmacists' Guide to Your Medicines*. New York: Ballantine, 1981.

*Wade, Carlson. *Miracle Protein*. West Nyack, NY: Parker Publishing Company, 1975.

*Weil, Andrew. *Health and Healing: Understanding Conventional and Alternative Medicine*. Boston: Houghton Mifflin, 1983.

*Whelan, Elizabeth M., and Stare, Frederick J., M.D. *Panic in the Pantry*. New York: Atheneum, 1975.

Williams, Roger J. *Nutrition Against Disease*. New York: Pitman Publishers, 1971.

*Winter, Ruth. *A Consumer's Dictionary of Food Additives*. New York: Crown, 1978.

*Yudkin, John. *Sweet and Dangerous*. New York: Peter H. Wyden, 1972.

Index